Deconstructing Yoga

A Secular Guide to Learning and Teaching

Julie Hanson &

Professor Lon Kilgore

ISBN-13:   978-0692348130
ISBN-10:   0692348131

Editor: Ashton J. Burchfield
Cover/Book Design: Killustrated – Azle – Texas – USA   killustrated.com
Publisher: Learning Hooks LTD – Glasgow – Scotland – UK learninghooks.com
                                      Killustrated – Azle – Texas – USA   killustrated.com

CONTENTS

"Frango ut patefaciam"
I break in order to reveal

Stephen J. Gould
quoting The Paleontological Society

My job in Deconstructing Yoga was to deliver written instruction into how to do and how to teach the asanas in a purely physical manner, while never losing sight of the over-bridging tenets of Yoga. Yoga does not have to be confined to Yoga studios. It can be used anywhere and everywhere, and it has a long history of being modified and changed to fit social, commercial, and practical needs. We have tried to create a book that is accessible to everyone. It is well known that many potential students are reticent to learn Yoga as its philosophies may be seen to conflict with their own belief systems. For many, the practices seem shrouded in mystery and they cannot discern which of the available systems of Yoga might fit them or indeed if the instruction they might receive will fulfill their purpose. There are also those who want to embark on a comprehensive exploration of yoga, starting with the foundation of all Yoga, the asanas. It is upon that initial establishment of the physical that all future development in Yoga is built.

- Julie Hanson

My job in Deconstructing Yoga was to dig deeply into the history, the science, and the practice of Yoga to frame up the asanas in an as objective and mythos free manner as possible. Every ancient practice that still exists today that accomplishes a change in human anatomy and physiology has an explanation of why it works. Although it is frequently ignored, there is a body of evidence surrounding the physical practice of Yoga and its effects on human musculoskeletal, cardiovascular, and neurocognitive function. We are not aware of a more comprehensive published review of the scientific literature exploring Yoga than what is presented in this book. Similarly, very few resources present a more even handed and relevant review of the history of Yoga's move into to the west than is included here. Whether in reviewing science, reviewing history, or in presenting the learning and teaching materials, we were careful to restrict our writings to what was known and to omit any belief sets that might bias the reader's interpretation and learned abilities.

- Lon Kilgore

SECTION 1 – UNDERSTANDING YOGA

"Blessed are the flexible, for they shall not be bent out of shape."

Anonymous

1 – UNTANGLING HISTORY

What is Yoga? Defining yoga is a difficult task, as there is a substantial mythos surrounding the word and practice. Many dozens of definitions can describe yoga, from two word phrases like "to join" to chapter long allegorical writings. If you look for commonalities and unifying threads between definitions you'll find that, in its broadest definition, yoga is a system of physical and mental skills used for self-development. The working definition used in this book has been further refined. However, before we are prepared to define yoga more specifically, we need to understand both the origins and the evolution of its nearly 4,000 year lifespan.

Yoga has obscure roots, putatively originating in the Vedic writings from between 1700 BC and 300 BC. In the older Gitā texts, yoga is divided into three branches. In the later Yoga Sūtras, it is presented in eight branches:

- Yama (ethics)
- Niyama (discipline)
- Asana (physical practice)
- Pranayama (breathing)
- Pratyahara (sensory withdrawal)
- Dharana (concentration)
- Dhyana (contemplation)
- Samadhi (ecstasy)

It is believed that in approximately 400 BC, two individuals named Patañjali codified the practice and teaching of yoga into the texts, the Yoga Sūtras, that would later be assimilated into many aspects of modern yoga (1). While the lineage of yoga as a theological pursuit is an ancient one, the emergence of the physical practice we recognize as yoga today did not begin until much later. There are no written records describing the asanas (postures) prior to the 11th century (2).

The next major works that affected the development and practice of modern yoga were the Goraksha Samhita by Yogi Gorakshanath (circa 11th-12th century), Haṭha Yoga Pradīpikā by Yogi Swatamarama (circa 15th century), the Shiva Samhita by an unknown author (circa 17th century), and the Gheranda Samhita by Yogi Gheranda (circa 17th century). Hatha yoga focused on the physical rather than the spiritual as in previous incarnations of yoga practice. While it is more physical, traditional hatha yoga, as derived from these writings, is a holistic practice that includes disciplines, postures, physical and mental purification procedures, ritual gestures, breathing, and meditation.

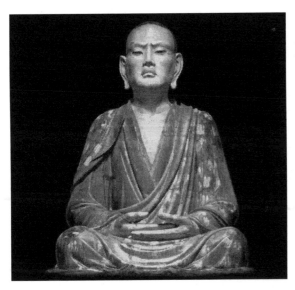

Figure 1-1. Virtually everyone who hears the word yoga associates it with eastern religious philosophy, often directly to meditation, as in this pose (photographed at the Nelson Atkins Museum, Kansas City, Missouri).

Mircea Eliade, who studied at the University of Calcutta from 1928 to 1931, was one of the first western academics to study yoga. He examined Indian religious practices, including yoga, as both an academic and a practitioner (3). Later becoming a professor at the University of Chicago, Eliade suggested that yoga incorporated diverse "spiritual and mystical" elements and that the practice transcended the physical body. This early description of yoga as a spiritual or trans-corporeal practice would color later perceptions of the discipline.

Most modern academics who have examined yoga similarly studied its spiritual elements instead of its physical aspects. The works of Feuerstein (4) and Wicher (5) independently concluded that yoga aimed to transcend consciousness and liberate oneself from bodily or worldly existence. Similarly, organizations that teach yoga instructors have also tended to adopt a definitive spiritual bias in their definitions and philosophies of yoga. The British Wheel of Yoga defines yoga as having "the aim of eventually achieving a direct encounter with or knowledge of the ultimate reality" (6). This type of definition persists globally, but is essentially too vague and subjective to be of satisfactory use in health practices or scientific investigation. Furthermore, it is ill-suited for use in discussions with western populations as it relies on the paranormal.

The belief that yoga is connected to the spiritual or metaphysical continues to persist. The New Age movement of the 1960's, characterized by younger groups adopting alternative approaches to traditional western culture, popularized eastern mysticism and the practice of yoga. There is a substantial contemporary population that is attuned and potentially receptive to the spiritual aspects of yoga; it is often suggested that there are as many as 50-75 million "new age-ers" in the USA. Regardless, for teaching purposes, especially for the beginning instructor, the physical practice of yoga without consideration of metaphysical aspects is fundamentally more appropriate to teach in general fitness and clinical environments. It is physical yoga, sans the more indefinable aspects of the spiritual, which allows objectivity, measurability, direction of programming, and goal setting.

A SYMBIOSIS WITH BRITAIN

Yoga's route to and influence by the UK is a surprising one. It developed there not from the calm and serene image the discipline is portrayed with today. Between the 14th and 17th centuries yogis were religious leaders with considerable political influence. Focused more on gaining worldly power than enlightenment, yogis and their disciples existed as substantial military units so commonly that by the 18th century there were hundreds of thousands of yogis employed as soldiers (7). This puts into context some of the names of postures used in yoga, like Warrior 1, 2, and 3 (the Sanskrit name Virabhadrasana translates roughly to fierce warrior). It is purported that the diminution of yoga's association in creating indigenous soldiers began with the prolonged British military occupation and control over the majority of South Asia after the Battle of Plassey (Jang e Palasi) in 1757.

The colonial presence of the British in India appears to have influenced the structure of Yoga. In a very thorough analysis of the history of the asanas of modern yoga (8), it was noted that there has been constant evolution and amalgamation in them. Oral history, indigenous practices, western gymnastics imported to India after the 18th century, wrestling training methods, and British military training exercises have all impacted the development of the physical practice of yoga (including the influence of the "father of modern yoga", Tirumalai Krishnamacharya). Kicking, punching, jumping, and rope drills were included in yoga training. It has further been suggested that yogis were often employed to lead physical training of British military units on the ground in India. These relatively modern findings demonstrate external influences, but do nothing to diminish the merit of the more ancient practices passed down through oral tradition; they simply indicate that yoga masters were ready to add effective practices to their teachings in order to better serve their philosophies and teaching needs. This also demonstrates that there was an informational flow both ways, from India to Britain and Britain to India. This was key to introducing yoga to the west.

For more than two centuries, the strong link between Britain and India and the resulting convenience of travel led a number of influential yogis to visit Britain and begin disseminating their teachings and influential British persons to travel to India in pursuit of enlightenment.

It is surmised here that as British influence became less desirable and the return to Indian nationalism more pronounced (re-assumption of indigenous practices and dress that had diminished due to western occupation), yoga teachings changed. While there seemed to be a return to a stronger focus on elements passed down by oral tradition, reversion to practices tracing to the military roots of the 17th century were not restored. Rather, in the 19th and 20th centuries, the current social and political philosophies— exemplified by the works of Vivekananda (1863-1902) and by Mahatma Ghandi (1867-1948)—imposed a more placid approach to yoga, the approach and body of teachings with which we are more familiar.

The Indian connection and the influence of acknowledged Yogis were vital to bringing yoga to Britain. On the other hand, two individuals that were indispensable to the cause were not devotees of yoga philosophy; rather, they were promoters of the physical practice. Mary Bagot Stack accompanied her military husband to India in 1912. While there she was taught yoga. In 1930, Mrs. Stack formed the Women's League of Health and Beauty (now the Fitness League), which attracted 166,000 women into its ranks and its practice of exercises based on yoga and dance within 7 years of its creation.

Another influential 20th century yoga teacher in Britain was Yogini Sunita, otherwise known as Bernadette Cabral. Cabral was born in India of English-Indian descent and in early adulthood worked in the Italian embassy in Bombay. In 1959 her family moved to Britain and she began her career of teaching relaxation and yoga (9). It was also in the 1940s and 50s that the UK physical culture magazine, Health & Strength, began to carry some content on yoga. This helped expose yoga to the world as a system of exercise.

A more formal presence of a yogi trained in the traditional master-mentor system that made his way to Britain was Bellur Krishnamachar Sundararaja Iyengar. His influence would extend from his arrival in Britain in 1952 until the present day. Another later influence from India came in 1973 in the form of Pattabhi Jois. Both of these individuals were trained by Tirumalai Krishnamacharya and they are associated with two distinct styles of yoga practiced in the west, Iyengar and Ashtanga yoga respectively.

IGNOBLE BEGINNINGS TO VORACIOUS CONSUMPTION – THE USA

The first American born yoga instructor was Pierre Bernard, born Perry Baker in Leon, Iowa in 1876. Humble origins in an Iowa-Missouri border town with a population of 820 belied the future of a person who would have a profoundly influential and negative effect on yoga for over 50 years. In 1889 Baker met and apprenticed under Sylvais Hamati, a hatha yoga teacher from Syria. Hamati also practiced hypnotism and dabbled in the occult. His teachings extended from yoga into sexual ritual and magic. It was during this association and the following move to San Francisco that Baker took on the name Pierre Bernard, presumably to add a continental flair to their marketing. Hamati and Bernard serviced elite clients for $100 (over $2000 in today's economy). While apparently a lucrative operation, the pair were ejected from San Francisco in 1906 and then from Seattle in 1909. The money finally stopped when Bernard was officially accused of a variety of offenses (use of magic, white slavery, soliciting blood oaths, and sexual exploitation of female devotees) and was ultimately convicted in a New York court for abduction and for impersonating a physician in 1910. Sensational headlines surged across the country, telling of the sordid case and legal proceedings. Although the final offenses resulted in only three months of jail time, irreparable damage had been done to the reputation of yoga and those who practiced or taught it. Yoga became considered a danger to women and society.

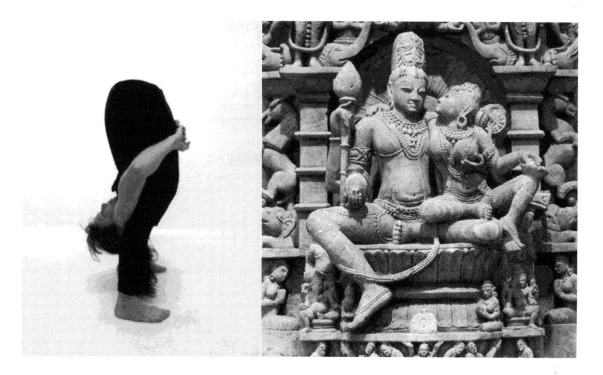

Figure 1-2. Yoga has had a historically difficult time with public perception. Frequently the public, the medical community, the media, and politicians identify Yoga as a form of contortionism attainable by a small elite few (left) or as an ancient set of sexual practices (right).

In 1947, yoga began a process of recovery via the classic American fascination with Hollywood. A high profile yoga teacher migrated to the USA. But Eugenie Peterson, better known as Indra Devi, was from Latvia, not India. She opened a Hollywood hatha yoga school to cater to the fitness and physical culturists who populated the southern California acting community. As every business enterprise knows, celebrity clientele often creates demand and profit through rapid and thorough marketplace penetration. Devi's practice flourished and her methods were committed to print in "Forever Young, Forever Healthy" (10). This particular book distanced the practice of yoga from the shadow of the mysticism and occult that Bernard had tainted Yoga with, towards the new yoga: yoga as a vivifying, health promoting activity. The dominance of presenting physical postures as content, rather than extensive philosophical discourses, was the first step towards easing yoga into the mainstream of exercise and health promotion.

As Hollywood actresses signed on to the practice, western attitudes towards yoga softened and yoga practices increased in number. In the 1950's, YWCAs and YMCAs began to deliver yoga sessions to their members. Such offerings from these Christian organizations speak strongly of the change in perception of yoga. Riding the current of this fresh perception came the suggestion that the physical aspects of the practice of yoga, divorced from yoga's spiritual and meta-physical beginnings, could form a viable and desirable system of exercise for western populations.

Shortly after Devi's success with those that appeared so often in front of Hollywood cameras, yoga itself made its on-camera debut on American TV. In 1970, Lilias Folan hosted and led a hatha yoga based exercise program on WCET, the Cincinnati Ohio affiliate of the Public Broadcasting System. Four years later, "Lilias, Yoga and You" was broadcast nationally and ran for 500 episodes and an impressive twenty five years, until 1999. Her program attracted much media attention and it was not uncommon for Lilias to teach and perform postures with the celebrity hosts of day and evening talk and variety shows in front of their millions of viewers. While many of her peers and predecessors contributed vitally to the development of western yoga, Folan is undoubtedly responsible for putting it in front of an entire nation.

Yoga was then poised to become a much larger and more accepted exercise system. Perhaps this potential would have been realized, had it not been for the influence of Dr. Thomas Cureton, Dr. Kenneth Cooper, and others, who had begun the quest of pushing aerobic exercise to the forefront of fitness and health promotion in the 1960s and 1970s. Jogging, without the perceived need for a trainer to facilitate exercise, coupled with the rise of dance-type aerobics, took center stage and rapidly sapped any progress of the further assimilation of yoga into the mainstream.

Although yoga had distanced itself from the paranormal in practice to an extent, the connection to hocus pocus remained seeded in the clinical professions. In his 1974 article in Canadian Family Medicine, Dr. Douglas Shatz discusses non-mainstream fitness methods, yoga prominent among them (11). His assessment portrays a negative bias but a seemingly begrudging acknowledgement of efficacy: "At the moment these techniques appear unscientific and spooky—but they work." That ability to change the physical body was again documented in medical literature in 1982. A paper by Andrews et al. in the British Medical Journal presented evidence that yoga could be used as a therapy for hypertension (12). Since those early medical publications, there has been mounting support for the use of yoga as a health and fitness intervention. A quick search of the National Library of Medicine's search engine (PubMed) using the search term "yoga" shows 1,749 clinical and scientific papers produced on the topic since 1964, with the vast majority of them, 1653, being published after 1990, and an astounding 1531 of these after 1998. The US National Institutes for Health created the National Center for Complementary and Alternative Medicine in 1998 as a structure to systematically investigate alternative medicine practices, including yoga. It appears from the latter number as though governmental and medical interests in the positive effects of yoga have spurred scientific investigations into its practice and outcomes. The results have largely been quite favorable; in fact, the current Director of this national research center, yoga practitioner Josephine Briggs, MD, writes about it on her "director's page", and in 2012 launched the Science of Yoga for Health and Well-Being effort (http:/nccam.nih.gov/health/yoga). The physical practices of yoga and their effects on fitness and health have become mainstream.

It's not just the governmental medical and scientific communities that are still moving yoga into a more mainstream position. The US Army uses the practice of yoga as part of the course of therapeutic treatment for combat induced post-traumatic stress disorder. On the flip-side, the US Army also uses yoga-derived methods (among others) to augment physical and mental function during Warrior Mind Training. It is clear that there are broad applications of yoga relative to health, fitness, and performance, even in the most hazardous workplace.

YOGA GROWS

It is relatively easy to demonstrate the growth of interest in yoga within the medical and scientific communities. Published scientific and medical professional position papers document the evolution of yoga from cult status to a growing scientific interest that is soon to become a widely-accepted exercise tool for health and fitness. However, documenting the acceptance of yoga within the general population is a little harder to do. There are numbers, but do these represent simple participation in yoga-like activities, participation in one of the variants of Hatha yoga, or do they reflect adoption of all or only some of the originally touted spiritual elements?

In the 1960s approximately 50,000 Americans exercised using yoga. By 1990 participation had risen to one million individuals, each training in general one to two times per week. In 1994, estimates suggested that there were six million regularly (and irregularly) engaging participants. Data for 2002 (four years after the formation of the

National Center for Complementary and Alternative Medicine) indicates an estimated 10 million participants. Participation continues to climb. Current statistics suggest that 15 million Americans practice yoga with some frequency with 72% of the participants being female. In Australia there are 1.6 million participants (90% female) and there are an estimated 500,000 in the UK. Anecdotal evidence in the UK suggests that, like Australia, about 90% of participants are female (13).

Despite the popular public image of Yoga as a spiritual and ascetic pursuit, nearly $3 billion is spent on instructors' salary annually. Approximately $5 billion is spent annually on yoga clothing and equipment. 71% of participants of yoga are university graduates and 44% earn more than $75,000 annually. The average participant will spend $1,800 annually on instruction and gear. Although these statistics imply that yoga participants have a fair amount of disposable income, yoga can be quite affordable. The fact that Wal-Mart, ASDA, Tesco, Myers, and more offer yoga mats and training apparel for purchase implies a grassroots demand for goods to support yoga participation and instruction services (13).

The history of yoga has always been linked to the improvement of the human physical condition. Yoga purists may consider modern yoga, which isolates the physical elements of training (asana), to be untrue to the original writings and philosophy of the discipline. However, the substantial cultural and intellectual evolution of yoga since the Vedic writings make this stance untenable. As fitness professionals, we are compelled to deliver physical instruction to improve fitness and promote health. The physical aspects of yoga practice reliably produce that result. Furthermore, the production of significant fitness improvements in our trainees through physical yoga practice catalyzes the resulting psychological benefits that the early sage's desired.

It should be relatively apparent that entwined in yoga is a very complicated system of belief and activity. Even when we consider Hatha yoga, the most common western form, there are numerous elements included beyond the purely physical acts of movement and holding postures. If we really want to recreate the practice of yoga into a form that directly addresses fitness promotion and the national health agenda, we need to change our approach. We need to utilize only the movements and postures and omit the ritualistic, spiritual, and metaphysical components included in the original writings. What remains is a system of low impact exercise that promotes balance, coordination and muscular fitness. For most commercial and clinical purposes this is a valuable set of results for the client or patient. These results simultaneously help fitness professionals or clinicians achieve their fitness, health and rehabilitation goals. The final result is a marketable fitness product accessible to everyone.

What we are doing is stripping yoga down to its bare, physical, essentials. To do this there is a small philosophical question we need to deal with; if we omit everything except the physical movements and postures from yoga, can we call it yoga?

This is a difficult question. A puritanical yogi might argue "No," as there are multiple limbs to yoga and without attention to all it is not truly yoga. However, since every expert yogi began in the physical realm of practice, we will argue "Yes."

In many ways, modern stretching exercises and body weight calisthenics are derived from yoga. In the exercise arena there are very few new things. Stretching-type movements have been part of exercise programs for likely as long as there have been humans. We can go back prior to the emergence of yoga and note that depictions of stretching appear in pre-Vedic Indian art of at least 5,000 years ago. Yogic writings formalized these practices into a system. Any time we stretch, we are doing something humans have been doing throughout recorded history. For yoga practice to have survived so long and to have affected sport, fitness, and health practice, it must have either worked towards achieving a goal or felt really good. Yoga can do both. When executed appropriately it will increase the range of motion around a joint and it can, in certain applications, provide a pleasurable sensation. What we will learn later is that we can program yoga training to improve metabolic function as well.

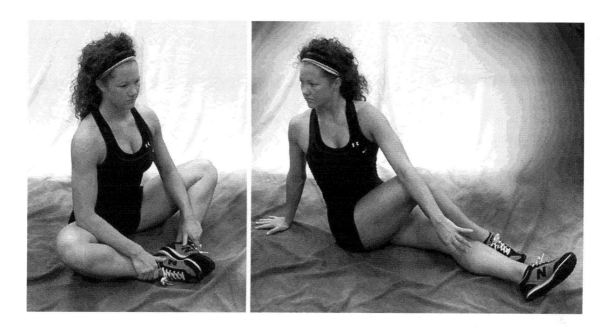

Figure 1-2. You see it every time you see exercise training sessions or sport practice, people doing variants of yoga practice ... stretching.

REFERENCES

1. Renou, L. On the Identity of the Two Patañjalis. In Navendra Nath Law. Louis de La Vallée Poussin Memorial Volume. 1940. Calcutta, India.
2. White, D.G. Sinister Yogis. 2009. University of Chicago Press, Chicago, IL.
3. Eliade, M. Yoga: Immortality and Freedom 2nd edition. 1969. Princeton University Press, Princeton, NJ. http://brihaspati.net/downloads/Yoga_Immortality_and_Freedom_Mircea_Eliade.pdf
4. Feuerstein, G. The Yoga Tradition: Its History, Literature, Philosophy and Practice. 1998. Hohm Press, Chino Valley AZ.
5. Wicher, I. The Integrity of the Yoga Darsana: A Reconsideration of Classical Yoga. 1998. State University of New York Press, Albany, NY.
6. Werner, K. Yoga, its Beginnings and Development. 1987. The British Wheel of Yoga, Farringdon, UK.
7. Pinch, W. Warrior Ascetics and Indian Empires. 2006. Cambridge University Press, Cambridge, UK.
8. Sjoman, N.E. The Yoga Tradition of Mysore Palace. 1996. Abhinav Publications, New Delhi.
9. Newcombe, S. Yoga and Ayurveda in Britain: 1950-1990, A Social History. 2008. PhD Dissertation, Faculty of History, University of Cambridge.
10. Devi, I. Forever Young, Forever Healthy. 1953. Prentice Hall, Saddle Ridge, NJ. (Reprinted in 2005 by Jaico Publishing, Mumbai India)
11. Shatz, D. Facing up to fitness. 1974. Canadian Family Medicine 20(4):70-72. http://www.ncbi.nlm.nih.gov/pmc/articles/PMC2274141/pdf/canfamphys00337-0072.pdf
12. Andrews, G. Hypertension: comparison of drug and non-drug treatments. 1982. British Medical Journal 284(6328): 1523-1526. http://www.ncbi.nlm.nih.gov/pmc/articles/PMC1498486/pdf/bmjcred00607-0023.pdf
13. Harris Interactive Service Bureau. (2012). Yoga in America – 2012. Sports Marketing Surveys USA.

2 – SCIENTIFIC ROOTS OF YOGA PRACTICE

As one can surmise from reading historical accounts of the origin and practice of yoga, it has often been lumped into the category of cult endeavors and popularly portrayed as having little or no scientific foundation in practice or effect. If one considers only the historical writings and their modern adaptations, it is easy to understand this criticism; however, when we fully examine the effects of physical yoga, the truth emerges. Physical yoga's inclusion into modern therapeutic medicine and its validation in scientific literature has ensured its place as a mainstream endeavor in improving health and combating disease. It has long been a given that Yoga promotes one's ability to relax (1) but it also improves quality of life in a number of ways (2). Regular participation in Yoga improves walking gait (3) and reduces both perceived pain (4) and inflammatory response (5). The positive health effects do not end there. Consistent practice improves blood pressure (6), reduces incidences of insomnia (7), improves joint function and decreases symptoms of osteoarthritis (8), improves diabetic status (9), and lowers cholesterol levels and other contributors to cardiovascular disease risk (10). If we are to truly be experts in the practice of yoga, not only do we have to understand how to do it and teach it, but we also have to understand the science behind its effects on fitness and health.

SCIENCE RISES FROM MYSTICISM

The early claims made about yoga practice range from the commonplace to the miraculous. In the Hatha Yoga Padipika, it is stated that yoga can neutralize poison, eliminate any disease, crush evil, and create immortality in its practitioners (11). Because Western researchers were interested in the nature of these claims and their philosophical or religious bases, most publications were in this area (along with extended academic debate on the original authors and creators of yoga's philosophical documents). Late 19th and early 20th century academic output on the subject was rare and, in general, quite esoteric, with little concern for applying the principles of yoga as a system of exercise.

The writings of the early masters stimulated great interest in the examination of the theoretical and philosophical nature of yoga, a favorite and fertile topic for both comparative religious studies and social studies. As early as 1827 there were attempts to translate the conceptual basis of yoga into a form understandable by the western academic [12]. Colebrooke's work, the first paper to directly evaluate the original Sanskrit texts, concluded that yoga was centered upon the mystic and fanatical rather than on coherent philosophical bases. Senart in 1900 [33] and Vallée Poussin in 1937 [14] published papers on the relationship and similar structure of the systems of meditation between Yoga and Buddhism.

Mircea Eliades was one of the most influential academics in this arena with numerous academic analyses of the history and philosophy of yoga published throughout his career:

- The Comparative History of Yoga Techniques, 1933
- Yoga: Essai sur les origines de la mystique indienne, 1936
- Techniques du Yoga, 1948
- Traité d'histoire des religions, 1949
- Le Chamanisme, 1951
- Patanjali et Yoga, 1962

For any exercise program to be considered valid and useful it must not only produce results, but also stand up to objective scientific scrutiny. The numerous influences on the academic development of physical education and physical culture during the mid-19th century contributed to an expansion of interest in physical health and fitness. Many ideas seemed well founded; some were innocuous. Some, like yoga, were seen with superstition and there was a clearly stated need for a "larger amount of the science of physiology with which to direct and extend the application" (15). However, it was not until the mid-twentieth century that more "scientific" studies began.

PHYSIOLOGICAL & FITNESS EFFECTS

Some of the first scientific papers on yoga were not about how the system worked but on some rather interesting capabilities of yogis:

> Case of acquired ability to suck liquid into the rectum and colon.
> Kjellberg S.R., et al., Nord Med. 44(27):1102-3, 1950

> Remarkable feat of endurance by a yogi priest.
> Vakil, R.J., Lancet 2(6643):871, 1950

Research that actually examined the effect of yoga on aspects of fitness emerged about the time of Indra Devi's publication of her best-selling book "Forever Young, Forever Healthy." The impact of the media and culture on scientific interest cannot be discounted. Without the entrepreneurs bringing yoga into the public eye, the ivory tower would never have noticed and become interested.

Once the novelty of the strange abilities of yogi had diminished, more robust examinations of the effects of yoga on human fitness began. An obvious starting point was consideration of the effects of yoga training on range of motion – since extreme joint flexibility was a commonly displayed ability of most master yogi. It was immediately assumed that the physical practices (asana) in which practitioners engaged induced improved flexibility, an assumption that was formalized in the scientific and clinical literature as early as 1964 (16). As mentioned earlier, this relationship of yoga postures with improved flexibility led to the postures being sanitized of their yoga association, stripped of their Sanskrit names and being included as stretching exercises for the general public, athletes, and clinical populations. The fact that this occurred half a century ago and the practice persists to date is heavily indicative of the perceived and actual benefits of yoga on range of motion. If it didn't work, most likely practitioners would have abandoned the practice long ago.

A frequently included aspect of Hatha yoga is the inclusion of respiratory training, in the form of controlled and restricted flow breathing (pranayama). There had been reports of yoga masters who could reduce respiratory rate by as much as 75% of normal. Such observations might suggest alterations in oxygen handling kinetics or metabolic processes, so this was of interest to exercise scientists seeking to understand the processes and limits of human physiology (17, 18, 19). Most changes seen in pulmonary function are small to moderate in magnitude and are generally explained by improved respiratory muscle control leading to improved vital capacity (20, 21).

Metabolic adaptation induced by yoga has been investigated (22) in order to determine if the system of exercise was sufficient to meet American College of Sports Medicine recommendations for exercise intensity. Yoga practice has been documented to be normally conducted at a level of effort below that required to meet such recommendations (23). While this observation is borne out by data demonstrating that cortisol (the catabolic hormone) actually diminishes in concentration (24) during a yoga workout – indicative that an adaptive stress may not be present – the changes in actual health-related fitness measures noted suggest an atypical mechanism of fitness improvement (25, 26, 27, 28, 29). Although the degree of effort involved and physiological outcome is variable depending on workout construction, the link of yoga practice to health status is robust. This link seems tied to a dose response, with higher participation frequencies producing larger results (30).

Part of the mixed bag of results for the metabolic cost of yoga and its small adaptive drive can be linked directly to the intended outcome of the yoga training employed. If the intent is to increase range of motion, induce relaxation or manage perceived pain (31), intensities must be, and are intentionally, low. To measure cardiovascular demand and outcomes with yoga routines intending to reduce stress or pain and to increase range of motion only is a flawed approach.

CARDIOVASCULAR EFFECTS

If the metabolic cost of yoga is purportedly too low to drive cardiovascular adaptation, how can it promote improved cardiovascular health as practitioners believe it does? Part of this question and explanation must be rooted not in mechanism but actual reports of improved cardiovascular function.

As with respiratory rate, early researchers acted upon anecdotes of master yoga practitioners often being reported to be able to reduce heart rate to such low levels that coma or death should have been a result (32). These observations and early works led to the concept that yoga practice could be used to reduce hypertension and such a relationship has been consistently explored for more than forty years (33, 34, 35, 36, 37).

If yoga can improve blood pressure status, might it follow that it can also affect the development of ischemic heart disease or coronary artery disease? This is a question that has been examined for decades with most studies demonstrating the small, but significant, effect of yoga in the reduction of signs indicative of cardiovascular disease risk. These beneficial effects include an improved blood lipid profile, reduced blood glucose, reduced body fat mass, and reduced oxidative stress (38, 39, 40, 41, 42, 43, 44).

If exercise intensity is too low to meet American College of Sports Medicine guidelines on exercise prescription, how does yoga generate its beneficial effects? It is quite possible that the practice of yoga exercises selectively activates neuromuscular or cardiovascular genes that in turn produce the protective effects noted. A direct effect on gene expression by yoga practice has been reported (45). In a study investigating gene regulation in blood lymphocytes it was noted that two genes were up-regulated within two hours of a yoga session (46). This data suggests that the mechanical activity of yoga exercises may be satisfactory, apart from any cardiovascular demand, to produce a gene regulatory response. These effects are similar to those seen in the heart where a single stretch of the myocardium produces an up-regulation of protective Heat Shock Protein 70 (47). These are changes that lie outside the traditional skeletal muscle adaptive pathways relative to metabolism and suggest that yoga is beneficial as an exercise modality even if it does not strongly affect aerobic metabolism.

ORTHOPEDIC EFFECTS

As mentioned earlier, yoga has always been associated with having complete or greater than normal range of motion around the joints. This capability to increase range of motion was seen to have potential therapeutic value very early on. The first mention of yoga relative to orthopedic health was in a 1962 opinion piece on the potential value of yoga as a physiotherapeutic intervention (48). A similar piece was published in 1977 (49). Specifically, yoga has been examined and determined to produce mild to moderate improvements in osteoarthritis, carpal tunnel syndrome and low back pain (50, 51, 52, 53, 54, 55, 56). It has also been seen to improve gait and stability in geriatric populations, both important aspects of quality of life and daily function (57, 58).

While improvements in joint motion and improved stability are not often considered architectural changes, improving hyperkyphosis (dowagers hump) is an architectural change in vertebral column architecture. A small scale study of 75 year old women with diagnosed hyperkyphosis improved, as evidenced by an over 0.5cm increase in standing height after a program of yoga training (59). Interestingly, other fitness measures, including body awareness and perceived health, also improved as a result of the training. It is apparent that the physical practice of yoga has positive orthopedic effects that include improved range of motion, a more stable and coordinated gait, and improvement in vertebral architecture.

NEUROCOGNITIVE EFFECTS

Early studies of the 1960's of yoga and brain function were not particularly complementary. Terms like "brain wash" and "mysticism" were used in the medical literature as the neural and cognitive effects were poorly understood and there was a general distrust remaining in regards to yoga masters and their ethics and results (60, 61). There were also attempts at establishing yoga as a para-psychological endeavor like hypnosis (62). However, a simultaneous exploration of the use of yoga as complimentary psychological and psychiatric therapy was emerging along with conjectures about the mechanism of proposed therapeutic outcomes (63).

As with cardiovascular and pulmonary investigations, early studies investigated neural functions in Indian yogis to determine if their neural function differed from normal populations (64). In fact, during the psychedelic sixties there was a boom in considering yoga as a psychiatric and psychoanalytic tool in the treatment of numerous psychiatric conditions (65, 66). Generally the relaxation effects of yoga were being espoused by physicians as a means to treat anxiety, stress, and insomnia, among others. In the hay days of the benzodiazepines (valium was released in 1963) there were 2.3 billion doses sold in 1978 and in the USA alone. Physicians were looking for a means of using fewer prescriptions to treat symptoms and yoga seemed to present a viable option. One author in 1972 implied that yoga mimicked the same outcomes as tranquilizers and in fact could be considered a tranquilizer (67). Thirty five years later it was noted that physical yoga practice increased the levels of gamma-aminobutyric acid (GABA) in the brain (68). Any time GABA concentrations increase, a reduction in anxiety and/or a perceived state of relaxation occurs. Another researcher demonstrated that 12 weeks of yoga induced a reduction in cerebral blood flow, also indicative of reduced stress and anxiety (69). So it appears that early anecdotal reports and opinions were warranted in this aspect.

The most modern research continues to investigate the beneficial effects of physical yoga practice on a variety of neurocognitive outcomes. Interestingly, it appears that as few as seven weeks of yoga training can improve academic performance, an effect likely mediated by a reduction in perceived stress (70). Another modern result suggested by new research is improvement of comfort in conditions of social stress and comfort with body image after completing a program of yoga training (71).

Depression is now also a target for examination where yoga is concern as studies focus on a potentially therapeutic response from yoga practice (72). While the relaxation effects of yoga may not be as relevant for the population who suffers from depression, the subjects in this study experienced a decrease in depression, and unique to yoga therapy, had a discernible reduction in attention focused on presumed sources of distress that led or contributed to depression.

Yoga can make you healthier and more fit in a number of ways. Though it won't make you run a sub-3 hour marathon or bench press three wheels on each end of the bar, it will improve your range of motion (or flexibility) around virtually any moveable joint in the body. It will also improve muscular control and body stability. If you are a beginning exerciser it will make you stronger and improve endurance. For yoga instructors, these things are all important to communicate to trainees so they understand what they stand to gain from participation. These parameters are easy to measure and as such are excellent measures to use to show trainees their progress. This progress breeds more regular participation and adherence to exercise and health practices.

Harder to measure objectively, but also important in today's stress-filled world, are the relaxation and anti-depressive effects of yoga. While the data does support that there are defined effects, it is possible that the trainee may not fully appreciate and communicate the perceived benefit in neurocognitive function for up to five years. This means that the physical practice and the resulting physical function improvements must be the focus in the early years of yoga training, since seeing those measurable benefits will aid in retaining the trainee in regular practice until the neurocognitive results are later realized.

Finally, one must understand that there is no clinical or scientific evidence that yoga can cure disease. It cannot cure the common cold. It cannot cure cancer. In the most liberal of consideration, it may aid in treating, not curing, some orthopedic conditions. With fact based practitioners, the truth and tangible results will sell and keep clients returning. Mythology and empty promises will not.

REFERENCES

1. Melville GW, Chang D, Colagiuri B, Marshall PW, Cheema BS. Fifteen minutes of chair-based yoga postures or guided meditation performed in the office can elicit a relaxation response. Evidence Based Complementary & Alternative Medicine. 2012 doi: 10.1155/2012/501986.
http://www.ncbi.nlm.nih.gov/pmc/articles/PMC3265094/pdf/ECAM2012-501986.pdf

2. Corey SM, Vizzard MA, Bouffard NA, Badger GJ, Langevin HM. Stretching of the back improves gait, mechanical sensitivity and connective tissue inflammation in a rodent model. PLoS One. 2012 7(1):e29831. doi: 10.1371/journal.pone.0029831.
http://www.ncbi.nlm.nih.gov/pmc/articles/PMC3253101/pdf/pone.0029831.pdf

3. Geyer R, Lyons A, Amazeen L, Alishio L, Cooks L. Feasibility study: the effect of therapeutic yoga on quality of life in children hospitalized with cancer. Pediatric Physical Therapy. 2011. 23(4):375-9. doi: 10.1097/PEP.0b013e318235628c.

4. Büssing A, Ostermann T, Lüdtke R, Michalsen A. Effects of yoga interventions on pain and pain-associated disability: a meta-analysis. Journal of Pain. 2012. 13(1):1-9. doi: 10.1016/j.jpain.2011.10.001.

5. Kiecolt-Glaser JK, Christian LM, Andridge R, Hwang BS, Malarkey WB, Belury MA, Emery CF, Glaser R. Adiponectin, leptin, and yoga practice. Physiology & Behavior. 2012. 5;107(5):809-13.

6. Agte VV, Jahagirdar MU, Tarwadi KV. The effects of Sudarshan Kriya Yoga on some physiological and biochemical parameters in mild hypertensive patients. Indian Journal of Physiological Pharmacology. 2011. 55(2):183-7.

7. Afonso RF, Hachul H, Kozasa EH, Oliveira Dde S, Goto V, Rodrigues D, Tufik S, Leite JR. Yoga decreases insomnia in postmenopausal women: a randomized clinical trial. Menopause. 2012. 19(2):186-93.

8. Chyu MC, von Bergen V, Brismée JM, Zhang Y, Yeh JK, Shen CL. Complementary and alternative exercises for management of osteoarthritis. Arthritis. 2011. 364319. doi: 10.1155/2011/364319.

9. Pandey A, Tripathi P, Pandey R, Srivatava R, Goswami S. Alternative therapies useful in the management of diabetes: A systematic review. Journal of Pharmacy & Bioallied Science. 2011. 3(4):504-12. doi: 10.4103/0975-7406.90103.
http://www.ncbi.nlm.nih.gov/pmc/articles/PMC3249697/

10. Innes KE, Selfe TK, Taylor AG. Menopause, the metabolic syndrome, and mind-body therapies. Menopause. 2008. 15(5):1005-13. doi:10.1097/01.gme.0b013e318166904e. http://www.ncbi.nlm.nih.gov/pmc/articles/PMC2810543/

11. Sing P. Hatha yoga pradipika. New Delhi, India: Sri Satguru Publications, 1979.

12. Colebrooke H. On the philosophy of the Hindus. Part 1: Sánkhya, 1827.

13. Senart É. "Bouddhisme et Yoga," Revue de l'histoire des religions, 42(3): 345-364, 1900.

14. de la Vallée Poussin L. "Le boudisme et le yoga de Patañjali," Mélanges chinois et bouddhiques. 1937. 5(1936-1937): 223-242.

15. Taylor GH. An Exposition of the Swedish Movement Cure. New York: Fowler and Wells, 1860.

16. Huddleston OL. Flexibility Exercises for Physical Fitness. Archives of Physical Medicine & Rehabilitation. 1964. 45:581-4.

17. Hollmann W, Mukerji GS, Spiegelhoff W. Metabolism, respiration and circulation in yoga exercises. Deutsche Medizinische Wochenschrift. 1956. 27;81(17):675-6.

18. Stănescu DC, Nemery B, Veriter C, Maréchal C. Pattern of breathing and ventilatory response to CO2 in subjects practicing hatha-yoga. Journal of Applied Physiology – Respiratory, Environmental, Exercise Physioliology. 1981. 51(6):1625-9.

19. Ray US, Pathak A, Tomer OS. Hatha yoga practices: energy expenditure, respiratory changes and intensity of exercise. Evidence Based Complementary & Alternative Medicine. 2011. 241294. http://www.ncbi.nlm.nih.gov/pmc/articles/PMC3135902/pdf/ECAM2011-241294.pdf

20. Bhole MV, Karambelkar PV, Gharote ML. Effect of yoga practices on vital capacity. (A preliminary communication). Indian Journal of Chest Diseases. 1970. 12(1):32-5.

21. Birkel DA, Edgren L. Hatha yoga: improved vital capacity of college students. Alternative Therapy, Health & Medicine. 2000. 6(6):55-63.

22. Clay CC, Lloyd LK, Walker JL, Sharp KR, Pankey RB. The metabolic cost of hatha yoga. Journal of Strength & Conditioning Researcb. 2005. 19(3):604-10.

23. Hagins M, Moore W, Rundle A. Does practicing hatha yoga satisfy recommendations for intensity of physical activity which improves and maintains health and cardiovascular fitness? BMC Complementary & Alternative Medicine. 2007. 7:40. http://www.ncbi.nlm.nih.gov/pmc/articles/PMC2219995/

24. Kamei T, Toriumi Y, Kimura H, Ohno S, Kumano H, Kimura K. Decrease in serum cortisol during yoga exercise is correlated with alpha wave activation. Perceptual Motor Skills. 2000. 90(3 Pt 1):1027-32.

25. Balasubramanian B, Pansare MS. Effect of yoga on aerobic and anaerobic power of muscles. Indian Journal of Physiological Pharmacology. 1991. 35(4):281-2.

26. Tran MD, Holly RG, Lashbrook J, Amsterdam EA. Effects of Hatha Yoga Practice on the Health-Related Aspects of Physical Fitness. Preventive Cardiology. 2001. 4(4):165-170.

27. Bhutkar MV, Bhutkar PM, Taware GB, Surdi AD. How effective is sun salutation in improving muscle strength, general body endurance and body composition? Asian Journal of Sports Medicine. 2011. 2(4):259-66.
http://www.ncbi.nlm.nih.gov/pmc/articles/PMC3289222/pdf/ASJSM-2-259.pdf

28. Tracy BL, Hart CE. Bikram yoga training and physical fitness in healthy young adults. Journal of Strength & Conditioning Research. 2013. 27(3):822-30.

29. Jeter PE, Cronin S, Khalsa SB. Evaluation of the benefits of a kripalu yoga program for police academy trainees: a pilot study. International Journal of Yoga Therapy. 2013. (23):24-30.
http://iayt.metapress.com/content/3x94511x3u47n0q5/fulltext.pdf

30. Ross A, Friedmann E, Bevans M, Thomas S. Frequency of yoga practice predicts health: results of a national survey of yoga practitioners. Evidence Based Complementary & Alternative Medicine. 2012.
http://www.ncbi.nlm.nih.gov/pmc/articles/PMC3425136/pdf/ECAM2012-983258.pdf

31. Boyle CA, Sayers SP, Jensen BE, Headley SA, Manos TM. The effects of yoga training and a single bout of yoga on delayed onset muscle soreness in the lower extremity. Journal of Strength & Conditioning Research. 2004. 18(4):723-9.

32. Wenger MA, Bagchi BK, Anand BK. Experiments in India on "voluntary" control of the heart and pulse. Circulation. 1961. 24:1319-25.

33. Datey KK, Deshmukh SN, Dalvi CP, Vinekar SL. "Shavasan": A yogic exercise in the management of hypertension. Angiology. 1969. 20(6):325-33.

34. Gopal KS, Bhatnagar OP, Subramanian N, Nishith SD. Effect of yogasanas and pranayamas on blood pressure, pulse rate and some respiratory functions. Indian Journal of Physiological Pharmacology. 1973. 17(3):273-6.

35. Patel C, North WR. Randomised controlled trial of yoga and bio-feedback in management of hypertension. Lancet. 1975.19;2(7925):93-5.

36. Andrews G, MacMahon SW, Austin A, Byrne DG. Hypertension: comparison of drug and non-drug treatments. British Medical Journal (Clin Res Ed). 1982. 22;284(6328):1523-6.

37. Hagins M, States R, Selfe T, Innes K. Effectiveness of yoga for hypertension: systematic review and meta-analysis. Evidence Based Complementary & Alternative Medicine. 2013. http://www.ncbi.nlm.nih.gov/pmc/articles/PMC3679769/

38. Tulpule TH, Shah HM, Shah SJ, Haveliwala HK. Yogic exercises in the management of ischaemic heart disease. Indian Heart Journal. 1971. 23(4):259-64.

39. Nespor K. Yoga and cardiovascular disease prevention. Casopis Lékaru Ceských. 1979. 16;118(11):333-5.

40. Dostálek C, Lepicovská V. Hathayoga-a method for prevention of cardiovascular diseases. Activitas Nervosa Superior (Praha). 1982. Suppl 3(Pt 2):444-52.

41. Bijlani RL, Vempati RP, Yadav RK, Ray RB, Gupta V, Sharma R, Mehta N, Mahapatra SC. A brief but comprehensive lifestyle education program based on yoga reduces risk factors for cardiovascular disease and diabetes mellitus. Journal of Alternative Complementary Medicine. 2005. 11(2):267-74.

42. Innes KE, Bourguignon C, Taylor AG. Risk indices associated with the insulin resistance syndrome, cardiovascular disease, and possible protection with yoga: a systematic review. Journal of the American Board of Family Practice. 2005. 18(6):491-519. http://www.jabfm.org/content/18/6/491.full.pdf

43. Gokal R, Shillito L, Maharaj SR. Positive impact of yoga and pranayam on obesity, hypertension, blood sugar, and cholesterol: a pilot assessment. Journal of Alternative & Complementary Medicine. 2007. 13(10):1056-7.

44. Yang K. A review of yoga programs for four leading risk factors of chronic diseases. Evidence Based Complementary & Alternative Medicine. 2007. 4(4):487-91. http://www.ncbi.nlm.nih.gov/pmc/articles/PMC2176145/

45. Saatcioglu F. Regulation of gene expression by yoga, meditation and related practices: a review of recent studies. Asian Journal of Psychiatry. 2013. 6(1):74-7.

46. Qu S, Olafsrud SM, Meza-Zepeda LA, Saatcioglu F. Rapid gene expression changes in peripheral blood lymphocytes upon practice of a comprehensive yoga program. PLoS One. 2013. http://www.ncbi.nlm.nih.gov/pmc/articles/PMC3629142/

47. Chang J, Wasser JS, Cornelussen RN, Knowlton AA. Activation of heat-shock factor by stretch-activated channels in rat hearts. Circulation. 2001. 10;104(2):209-14.

48. Prerez Bocanegra R. Yoga and physiotherapy. Medecine tropicale (Madr). 1962. 38:273-82.

49. Levitz L. Yoga and rehabilitation. American Archives of Rehabilitation Therapy. 1977. 25(1):11-6.

50. Garfinkel MS, Schumacher HR Jr, Husain A, Levy M, Reshetar RA. Evaluation of a yoga based regimen for treatment of osteoarthritis of the hands. Journal of Rheumatology. 1994. 21(12):2341-3.

51. Kolasinski SL, Garfinkel M, Tsai AG, Matz W, Van Dyke A, Schumacher HR. Iyengar yoga for treating symptoms of osteoarthritis of the knees: a pilot study. Journal of Alternative & Complementary Medicine. 2005. 11(4):689-93.

52. Haaz S, Bartlett SJ. Yoga for arthritis: a scoping review. Rheumatic Disease Clinics of North America. 2011. 37(1):33-46. http://www.ncbi.nlm.nih.gov/pmc/articles/PMC3026480/pdf/nihms-252756.pdf

53. Telles S, Naveen KV, Gaur V, Balkrishna A. Effect of one week of yoga on function and severity in rheumatoid arthritis. BMC Research Notes. 2011. 12;4:118. http://www.ncbi.nlm.nih.gov/pmc/articles/PMC3083351/pdf/1756-0500-4-118.pdf

54. Garfinkel MS, Singhal A, Katz WA, Allan DA, Reshetar R, Schumacher HR Jr. Yoga-based intervention for carpal tunnel syndrome: a randomized trial. JAMA. 1998. 11;280(18):1601-3.

55. Hudson S. Yoga aids in back pain. Australian Journal of Advanced Nursing. 1998. 5(9):27.

56. Galantino ML, Bzdewka TM, Eissler-Russo JL, Holbrook ML, Mogck EP, Geigle P, Farrar JT. The impact of modified Hatha yoga on chronic low back pain: a pilot study. Alternative Therapy, Health & Medicine. 2004. 10(2):56-9.

57. DiBenedetto M, Innes KE, Taylor AG, Rodeheaver PF, Boxer JA, Wright HJ, Kerrigan DC. Effect of a gentle Iyengar yoga program on gait in the elderly: an exploratory study. Archives of Physical Medicine and Rehabilitation. 2005. 86(9):1830-7.

58. Hart CE, Tracy BL. Yoga as steadiness training: effects on motor variability in young adults. Journal of Strength & Conditioning Research. 2008. 22(5):1659-69.

59. Greendale GA, McDivit A, Carpenter A, Seeger L, Huang MH. Yoga for women with hyperkyphosis: results of a pilot study. American Journal of Public Health. 2002.

92(10):1611-4.

http://www.ncbi.nlm.nih.gov/pmc/articles/PMC1447294/pdf/0921611.pdf

60. Mukherjee DR. Yoga. Yogic...brain-wash. Psychology and neurology. Indian Medical Journal. 1961. 55:106-13.

61. Hayman M. Science, Mysticism and Psychopharmacology. California Medicine. 1964. 101:266-71.

62. http://www.ncbi.nlm.nih.gov/pmc/articles/PMC1515670/pdf/califmed00076-0033.pdf

63. Das JP. Yoga and hypnosis. International Journal of Clinical & Experimental Hypnosis. 1963. 11:31-7.

64. Ramamurthi B. Yoga-an explanation and probable neurophysiology. Journal of the Indian Medical Association. 1967. 48(4):167-70.

65. Wenger MA, Bagchi BK. Studies of autonomic functions in practitioners of Yoga in India. Behavioral Science. 1961. 6:312-23.

66. Malhotra JC. Yoga and Psychiatry: A Review. Journal of Neuropsychiatry. 1963. 4:375-85.

67. Neki JS. Yoga and psychoanalysis. Comprehensive Psychiatry. 1967. 8(3):160-7.

68. Arbe A. That new tranquilizer called yoga. Medical Times. 1972. 100(9):170.

69. Streeter CC, Jensen JE, Perlmutter RM, Cabral HJ, Tian H, Terhune DB, Ciraulo DA, Renshaw PF. Yoga Asana sessions increase brain GABA levels: a pilot study. Journal of Alternative & Complementary Medicine. 2007. 13(4):419-26.

70. Cohen DL, Wintering N, Tolles V, Townsend RR, Farrar JT, Galantino ML, Newberg AB. Cerebral blood flow effects of yoga training: preliminary evaluation of 4 cases. Journal of Alternative & Complementary Medicine. 2009. 15(1):9-14.
http://www.ncbi.nlm.nih.gov/pmc/articles/PMC3155099/pdf/acm.2008.0008.pdf

71. Kauts A, Sharma N. Effect of yoga on academic performance in relation to stress. International Journal of Yoga. 2009. 2(1):39-43.
http://www.ncbi.nlm.nih.gov/pmc/articles/PMC3017967/

72. Hafner-Holter S, Kopp M, Günther V. Effects of fitness training and yoga on well-being stress, social competence and body image. Neuropsychiatry. 2009. 23(4):244-8.

73. Kinser PA, Bourguignon C, Whaley D, Hauenstein E, Taylor AG. Feasibility, acceptability, and effects of gentle hatha yoga for women with major depression: findings from a randomized controlled mixed-methods study. Archives of Psychiatric Nursing. 2013. 27(3):137-47.

"It's only work if somebody makes you do it."

Calvin
Sam Watterson's *Indispensable Calvin and Hobbes*

3 – YOGA, MOBILITY AND ENDURANCE

One of the fundamental physical adaptations resulting from yoga practice is a change in mobility. Mobility can be defined as the ability to move the body and its constituent parts in a variety of directions and carry out both simple and complex motor tasks. Very simply stated, mobility is movement. Mobility is an important—but under-attended—element of fitness, as stable, controlled, and coordinated movement within our occasionally unstable and frequently unpredictable home, work, and play environments is important for adequate function and living.

Mobility is likely the most complicated element of overall fitness as it is a combination of joint range of motion and motor abilities: agility, balance, and coordination. If we consider things from a subjective, trendy perspective, mobility is, in essence, a state of being. On the other hand, we will objectively describe that state as: the possession of the required physical properties to move as needed within one's own circumstances.

Mobility varies considerably across the life span and is generally correlated with high amounts of exercise or physical activity. As the frequency, intensity, and duration of exercise increases, so too does mobility. Exercise improves mobility and advancing age diminishes it. With increasing age, mobility tends to decrease due to loss of range of motion around numerous joints (1) and also due to a slowly developing decrement in the processing of sensory information, a vital component of motor skills (2). These observations are important for yoga instructors as the majority of students whom they will teach will be over 35 years of age.

While mobility decrements seem to be somewhat inevitable, a voluntary lack of exercise or physical activity will hasten these issues. This creates a vicious cycle: aging reduces range of motion and sensory information processing, failure to remain active in advanced age induces further reductions in mobility, and range of motion is reduced further as aging and inactivity continue. But it is not just older populations who must concern themselves with mobility; a sedentary lifestyle reduces mobility in even the youngest of populations. Only the rate of decay is different.

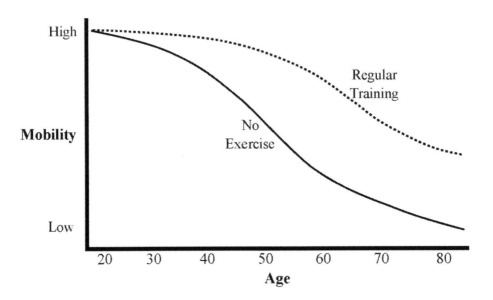

Figure 3-1. The decline in mobility with advancing age. Although the solid line represents total mobility, it can be accurately used to illustrate both range of motion and motor ability decline over the life span. The dotted line demonstrates the effect of regular exercise training over time, a drastically reduced decline in mobility (retention of mobility for more of the life span).

This is where a problem arises. The concept of mobility is relatively complicated, not necessarily because the definition given earlier is invalid, but because of the relative lack of data and standards associated with mobility. Much of the problem stems from inadequate definitions and incorrect usage of the terms associated with mobility.

As there is presently an absence of mobility standards available for use by fitness professionals and trainees, it is nearly impossible to know how much mobility any one person should possess, other than that person simply being able to complete their desired activities or movements. The stereotypical image of Indian yogis in positions of extreme contortion does little to provide practitioners or the public with a viable understanding of mobility. Many modern instructors contribute to the problem with their attempts to obtain extreme range of motions themselves and then to push the notion that an extreme range of mobility is desirable as a training outcome for all trainees. If students do not achieve it, the student is considered to have failed in obtaining fitness and health – hardly a rewarding experience for students. What is needed is an objective means for measuring mobility and then categorizing it.

Norms and standards are available for some aspects of mobility. The term "norm" here denotes what the average person is capable of. We know that the average person is not fit, so norms have limited validity and utility as a reference for determining how fit or mobile someone is or should be (3). Standards, on the other hand, are approximations of what would be expected of a trainee's performance in certain situations, and as such they may summarize the desirable amount of mobility for a given task. There are, for example, standards for range of motion and synchrony of movement (coordination) for an effective golf swing (4). Striking a golf ball requires a certain magnitude of range of motion and, as anyone who has ever swung a driver will tell you, coordination. Within sport there are many similar and defined examples, but for general fitness and health it is not clear how much of any component of mobility is needed. In yoga practice there is a similar lack of guidance available. There is little scientific or clinical evidence to indicate that a person who can reach eight inches past his toes is any more fit, in the global sense, than a person who can only reach the top of his toes. So are a prima ballerina's or a yogi's joints more fit and healthy than the average exerciser? Without clear definitions and standards we cannot make concrete statements one way or the other.

In addition to lacking useful mobility standards, the current lexicon of exercise terms used by the fitness community has seen "mobility" become synonymous with pre-habilitation, rehabilitation, and the use of various recovery modalities. While mobility does work in this context, there is something here at odds with fitness gain. In this context, restorative exercises and therapies are being used to return an injured or diseased joint system to health and the use of prophylactic exercises are being used to potentially prevent injury, NOT improve fitness. The only valid uses of "prehab" and "rehab" methods, when used in conjunction with an appropriate training program, are as an aid in the restoration of lost mobility.

This restorative application of clinical mobility training is not appropriate for healthy and active populations, except in cases of absolute physical inactivity in beginning trainees, or in more advanced trainees who have used a (or multiple) training program(s) that neglected mobility as an integral feature.

What is presented within these pages is an approach, using physical yoga practice, to put trainees on a correct training path that addresses mobility from the onset. Range of motion, agility, balance, and coordination are all integrated herein.

RANGE OF MOTION

An essential component of training to enhance mobility is working to develop an appropriate range of motion in the joint systems throughout the body. Yoga training excels at increasing range of motion.

Range of motion, as we specifically define it here, is possession of the ability to move a joint fully between its anatomical limits, proximal and distal. Those limits are generally set by the bony architecture of a joint but there are other normally active anatomical limitations. Think of the elbow. At complete extension, it is limited by the olecranon of the ulna being seated in the olecranon fossa of the humerus. The bone on bone contact sets one limit in the range of motion. The limitation at the other end is the contact of the surface of the forearm with the front of the upper arm when the elbow is flexed. This tissue on tissue inhibition of movement sets the second limit for elbow range of motion. Anything that limits or prevents these two conditions from occurring inhibits range of motion. The big meaty arm of an NFL offensive lineman or a prop in rugby will have, by virtue of the amount of muscle tissue present, a smaller range of motion during flexion than a waifish runway model or an elite marathoner. Regardless of the absolute degrees of range of motion here, the range of motion is "complete" as long as it is only limited by architectural structure.

Because bony structure is only mildly modifiable, within this context it is not a significant concern. Therefore, in application, range of motion can be considered the ability of the tissues surrounding a joint and the muscles that act upon a joint to contract and extend sufficiently to allow both passive or active movement completely through all joint angles within the joint's anatomical limits.

Flexibility is frequently used synonymously with range of motion. Good flexibility, the possession of a complete range of motion around the major joints—ankles, knees, hips, shoulders, elbows, and wrists—can be beneficial to one's ability to function effectively in training, sport, work, and daily life. A properly designed yoga program will increase an individual's range of motion by intelligent incorporation of exercise postures that require movements through complete ranges of motion. This is specifically the reason for insistence on correct technique and progression during every training session. It is also why postures have definite start and stop positions, to ensure complete range of motion is carried out with each repetition, movement, and posture.

Not everyone who starts a fitness program will possess even an average range of motion around all of the important joints. Instructors must be capable of assessing range of motion and adapting postures to meet individual needs. Furthermore, they must be capable of designing training sessions that move individuals through intuitive and intelligently selected series of postures to create improvements in mobility.

IMPROVING RANGE OF MOTION

As we have already learned, some of humanity's earliest writings, the Indian Vedas some 4000 years ago, described yoga. Also, we know that the idea for "stretching" is largely derived from yoga. While the practice of yoga is perceived as unfamiliar by the public, they are highly familiar with its derivative, stretching. This is not a new development. One of Edward Muybridge's 19th century motion pictures, which were the very first movies, was of a person doing a brief stretching exhibition. Stretching is a very familiar exercise concept to almost all people. They have done it in PE, done a semblance of it in the morning when they wake-up, they have even watched their dog or cat do it. Athletes pay attention to it and ballet dancers live and die by it.

In this context, yoga is a well-known and primary technique used to improve the state of one's flexibility, or, in other words, to increase the range of motion of a joint or set of joints. The specific exercises used are specific to and develop only the range of motion of the muscles and joints that perform the exercise. This means that each yoga posture or movement is specific to the muscles and joints recruited during that posture or movement. There is no one single posture or movement that works for all purposes and all joints.

The degree of range of motion, or flexibility, needed around a given joint is task specific; it is purpose driven. Prior to creating a yoga training program, the individual's ability to assume postures and move between positions must be assessed. This can be done by simply observing the joint angles the individual is able to attain during their first yoga session. If possible, a record of limitations should be made. This can provide notes of needed adaptations or starting points for the individual and a useful means of determining range of motion improvement.

In virtually every yoga posture and the movement of the body into that posture, there are multiple joints involved. It is a common occurrence that an individual may demonstrate excellent flexibility in one region of the body and poor flexibility, or stiffness, in other areas. It is incumbent on the yoga instructor to be able to determine where the limitation in range of motion occurs. Is it proximal or distal? Which muscle or muscles are the limiting elastic elements? This is why a functional knowledge of anatomy is quite useful in the practice of yoga instruction. Without that knowledge, one might be misidentifying limitations and approaching correction inappropriately by working on the wrong muscle groups.

"Stiff", as used above, is another interesting casual term that will be heard and used in conversation. In general, stiff means "resistant to bending," so it is actually a suitable descriptor only for conditions where full flexion of a joint is not achievable; it is not suitable for describing an inability to completely extend a joint. Flexibility is the more comprehensive layman's term.

Most people, trainees, coaches, clinicians, and media all assume that flexibility is an essential element of health and performance. However, the Healthy People 2020 national goals statement from the U.S. Department of Health and Human Services does not include a specific recommendation for inclusion of flexibility exercises (the objective was archived) as part of any exercise program. However, in the document, the authors did note a correlational importance between stretching and good health. This connection between stretching and health is based on a few biological observations: (A) Movement of a joint through a full range of motion creates pressure differences within the joint capsule that drives nutrients from the synovial fluid toward the cartilage of the joint. (B) Since cartilage lacks its own blood supply, the chondrocytes (the cells that produce cartilage) depend on diffusion of oxygen and nutrients from the synovial fluid for adaptation to occur. (C) This pressure-aided-fluid movement enhances diffusion and results in more viable chondrocytes. This series of events forms the basis for the assumption that stretching correlates with joint health. As yoga is the more systematic and effective parent of stretching, we can expect this correlation to be applicable to yoga trainees.

To understand how yoga affects range of motion, we need to look at the structure of a joint (figure 3-3). The range of motion around a joint or joints is a reflection of the extensibility and elasticity of the soft tissues at that joint and this in large part determines the extent and direction of any possible movement. A basic understanding of human anatomy is important in understanding the principles of yoga and its effect on range of motion. The nature and direction of movement at a joint is determined by the shapes of the bony surfaces that articulate at the joint. There are a number of different types of joints, classified by bony structure, with certain types allowing for greater magnitude and direction of movement than others. For example, the circular surface of the ball-and-socket joint of the hip allows considerably more movement, including movement to the side (adduction and abduction), forward and backward (flexion and extension), rotating in and out (internal and external rotation), and circumduction (swinging the leg in a big circle). Contrast that range of motion to that of the hinge joint that we know as the elbow. The elbow has a much more restrictive construction that limits movement to primarily forward and backward (flexion and extension). Knowing the anatomical limits of mobility allows us to qualitatively assess range of motion.

The properties of connective tissue (tendons and ligaments) and muscle affect range of motion. The extent of movement available at any joint is determined not only by the bony anatomy, type, and shape of the joint, but also by the ligaments, tendons, and muscles that attach to, stabilize, or cross the joint.

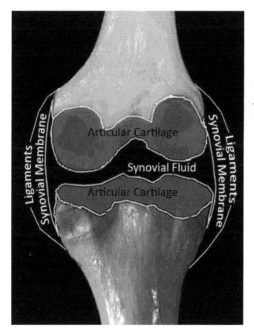

Figure 3-3. The basic structural elements of a joint. Note the cartilage and synovial fluid surrounding the bony structures of the bone.

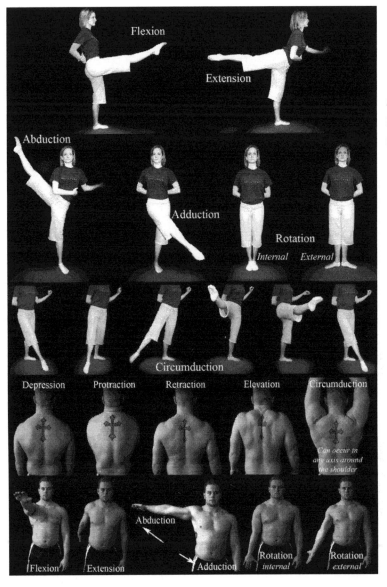

Figure 3-4. Examples of range of motion at the hip and shoulder.

Ligaments are tough and rather inelastic bands of connective tissues that connect bone to bone in order to create a joint. They provide rigidity and stability to the joint and a means to restrict excessive motion of the joint, a safeguard to dislocation. Tendons are also fibrous bundles of connective tissue; however, tendons connect muscle to bone. In general one muscle with a tendon at each end is attached to two different bones.

Muscles are collections of specialized cells that are contractile and, important to the issue of range of motion, are also somewhat extensible and elastic. To use a rope analogy, ligaments are built like caving ropes—with very little stretchability; tendons are like climbing ropes which only possess enough stretchability to add a little safety cushion in a fall; and muscles are like bungee cords that possess a great deal of stretchability. During movement, muscles and tendons are both loaded at the same time. Thus, when a joint is stretched, a muscle (or set of muscles) is stretched. Our primary target in efforts to improve range of motion is the muscle, as it holds the greatest potential for improvement. We do not want to make tendons more extensible. The job of the tendon is to transfer force from the muscle to the bone and if we make it more stretchable, we have decreased the ability of the tendon to transfer force.

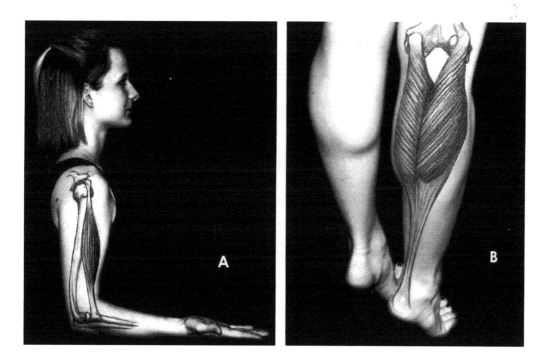

Figure 3-5. The tendon of a muscle attaches the muscle fibers to the bone (A – Bicep to radius and humerus, and B – Calf muscles to heel and femur), allows transmittance of contractile forces, and allows movement to occur.

Any muscle that crosses or is adjacent to a joint, basically any muscle that acts to move or stabilize a joint, directly influences flexibility. Generally, muscles involved with human movement are connected as pairs that have opposite movement actions. Given any movement, there is a muscle (or muscle group) that contracts to produce the movement. This is the agonist. Opposing the agonist, often on the opposite side of the joint, is a muscle (or group of muscles) that creates the opposite movement when contracted. This is the antagonist. When an antagonist muscle is contracted with equal force to the agonist, a static equilibrium between the agonist and antagonist is produced that yields no movement. It can also attempt to contract (but not actually shorten) and fractionally resist the movement driven by the agonist. In this movement the antagonist is undergoing an eccentric muscle action, generating force at the same time it is being stretched. This is one of the ways we control acceleration and deceleration during movement. This is also important in exercise as the amount of force generated to drive the movement can be either hampered or facilitated by the degree of relaxation (or non-recruitment) of the antagonist muscle(s). The more an antagonist muscle yields, the less energy it spends overcoming its resistance to the intended movement. Yoga training may assist in learning how to turn off the recruitment of antagonist muscles. Working to increase the range of motion around the joint teaches the muscles how to turn off, or at least dampen, the reflexes that activate antagonist muscles. This is germane to range of motion, as it may be limited, regardless of the amount of training invested, if the antagonist muscles are not capable of relaxation during agonist action. There may also be a negative effect on range of motion if there is a lack of coordination between contraction of the agonist muscle and relaxation of the antagonists. It is not surprising, therefore, that individuals with poor coordination, or an inability to relax the antagonist muscles, may have a low rate of range of motion improvement.

Range of motion can be measured in a variety of ways, but most commonly it is measured as a limit of rotation or movement through a specific range of motion with a static flexibility test. Clinically there is great interest in performing static range of motion testing of areas of the body that tend to lose range of motion with age and inactivity, such as the lower back (lumbar region) or the hamstring muscle group of the back of the legs. One of the most common range of motion assessments to measure flexibility in the low back region, in use clinically and commercially, is the "sit-and-reach test". The premise for such testing is a putative correlation between poor performance on the test and a higher incidence of low back pain (5, 6). Interestingly, sit-and-reach test scores are reflective of hamstring flexibility, NOT lower back flexibility (think about the anatomy of the hip and the movement tested). As such, published "sit-and-reach" norms may only be useful in the identification of individuals at the extremes of inflexibility who may be at higher risk for injury. There is not enough data available to provide specific static flexibility guidance other than identification of "normal" range of motion. Fitness professionals must also remember that, in measuring flexibility, attention to testing details is necessary. Static flexibility scores that are subjective, like "can you touch your toes?" are hugely affected by individual anatomical structure. An individual with longer arms and shorter torso will be able to accomplish the toe-touch task with a smaller range of motion than an individual with shorter arms and longer torso. There is also the psychological issue of individual differences in pain perception and tolerance during testing. Some individuals will stop at the first twinge of discomfort; others will drive more deeply into their pain threshold.

One thing that must be considered and attended to by yoga instructors is tracking range of motion improvements. There must be a means of identifying and progressing the degree of stress applied during postures and the movement between them. Principles of overload and progression are active here, as they are with any other exercise or fitness element, and must be applied to the use of yoga to improve range of motion.

PHYSIOLOGY OF RANGE OF MOTION IMPROVEMENT

For range of motion to be increased, the antagonist muscle or muscle groups must be stretched and held beyond normal resting lengths. This is why there is always a "hold" phase associated with every yoga posture.

It is relevant to interject a simple physical and biological reality here, although there are many commercial exercise systems that claim to make a muscle longer—this is, in fact, impossible without some relatively radical surgery. Muscle A is attached to bone B and bone C. There is nothing that any exercise can do to increase the distance between points B and C. This means a muscle cannot get longer in response to any exercise stimulus. The notion that a muscle gets longer with training comes from the observation of individuals with incomplete range of motion. When range of motion increases, the assumption for the uninformed practitioner is that the muscle added length. If this was the case there would be added mass (bodyweight) that accompanies any increase in range of motion. This is not supported by any scientific literature. What occurs is that the antagonistic muscles become more compliant. They resist movement to the anatomical limits less, and range of motion is improved. This increased range of motion is erroneously assumed to be muscle elongation. The muscle has always been this length; now, its function has simply been facilitated to allow full range of motion.

When a muscle is stretched, lengthened from its resting postural state, there is a reflex, the stretch reflex that acts to resist the stretch. Nervous receptors called muscle spindles contain several small "intrafusal" muscle cells that are tucked away inside and are parallel to regular or "extrafusal" muscle cells. They provide information regarding muscle length to the nervous system. Specifically, they detect the rate of change in length and report the information to the central nervous system. When a muscle is stretched, the body attempts to retain homeostasis, or, in this situation, posture. These sensory receptors in the muscle-tendon system send signals to the sensory neurons, nerves that detect environmental changes. These neurons further signal another set of neurons, motor neurons, to initiate the contractile process and shorten the muscle. Here is where proper exercise technique comes into play. If the movement into a yoga posture is carried out too quickly, this reflex fires, induces a counter-contraction in the stretched muscle, and restricts initial efforts and progress towards attaining movement through the complete range of motion. However, if the movement occurs more slowly and is held over time, the reflex is not strongly invoked, and any vestigial reflex that does occur will subside in a few seconds and allow the muscle to be stretched more fully towards its anatomical limits. The presence of this reflex explains why it is important to slowly apply and hold a yoga posture for no less than a period of 10-30 seconds. More quickly applied attempts to stretch or shorter duration posture holds are limited by the opposing action of the stretch reflex and defeat progress in enhancing range of motion.

Another receptor active in muscle is the Golgi tendon organ. Golgi tendon organs (commonly referred to as GTOs) are located within the transition area where muscle cells phase out and tendons phase in where they monitor tension. High forces applied to a muscle stimulate these receptors and provide an inhibitory reflex. This reflex would potentially be active only if there were fast, ballistic attempts at moving into differing postures. The normal and accepted method of yoga posture attainment and transition does not invoke this reflex. If it does, you are doing it wrong.

A slowly applied stretch of muscles creates less reflex contraction by way of muscle spindles and GTOs. If done slowly, muscle length changes do not invoke reflex contraction of the stretched muscle or muscles (myotactic reflex). It is unlikely that all reflex activation can be avoided, but as the posture is held, any residual stretch reflex present will abate and tension in the muscle decrease as the position is held over time. Most of this decrease in tension, or resistance to stretch, occurs in the first 10 seconds. As more repetitions of the posture are done, the tension curves, or how fast the resistance diminishes, lower. This is why not one but multiple repetitions of a yoga posture are recommended and included in yoga sessions.

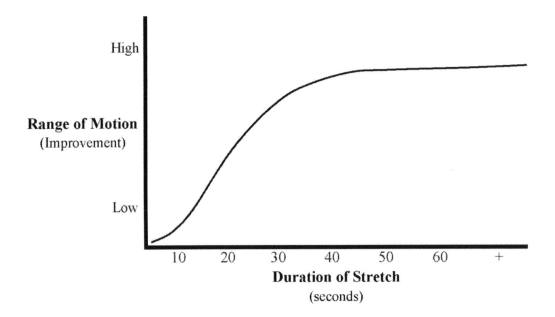

Figure 3-6. Benefits in range of motion begin with holds of about ten seconds and are maximized by about 30 seconds. Holding a posture for 60 seconds or more offers minimal additional increase in range of motion over much shorter durations. However, it may have an endurance effect.

Although there is a powerful neural component of employing yoga for improved range of motion, several other factors may affect range of motion and the body's response to yoga. Some factors are unavoidable. Age, presence of disease, previous injury to the muscle or joint, and the presence of scar tissue are all non-alterable. There are two extrinsic factors that are under individual control: (A) temperature, both environmental and body, and (B) muscle strength imbalance.

The former issue is an easy concept to grasp. As muscle temperature rises, elasticity increases. As extensibility of the muscle increases, range of motion at any joint around which that muscle is active improves. This is one of the concepts behind "hot yoga," better range of motion from being in a hot room. The opposite can also happen. As environmental and muscle temperature drops, flexibility decreases. This relationship may also explain why you feel stiffer in cold weather and why the cold has a negative influence on range of motion and response to stretching. Interestingly there is little evidence to support the concept that hot yoga is any more effective at improving range of motion **over time** than standard room-temperature yoga (7).

The second alterable factor is related to the ratio of strength between an agonist and antagonist muscle or group of muscle. The strength of the muscles on either side of the joint, or in some cases adjacent to the joint, affects its range of motion. Ideally, around each joint, the opposing muscles create a natural balance that allows the joint to move through its entire range of motion, from anatomical limit to anatomical limit. It must be understood that the natural balance referred to here is not a 50/50 balance between agonist and antagonist; it is simply the amount of strength required to maintain normal posture at rest, during movement, and under load. If an exercise program includes work in all relevant directions around a joint, an imbalance does not occur (remember, natural does not imply equal). Let us consider the shoulder here and use the easy example of weight training. If we do Presses, Dips, Bench Presses, and Rows, we have placed a balanced set of directional movement stresses on the joint and have thus limited the potential of an agonist or antagonist being disproportionately stronger. Unfortunately, this is often not the programming case in the modern fitness arena.

The use of machines and isolation exercises create an environment where it is easy to omit relevant musculature from a workout. This means that one muscle or set of muscles becomes weak relative to the opposing set. In this case, joint range of motion may be compromised. A common example of such an imbalance is found between the anterior and posterior shoulder muscles. Most recreational weight trainees and beginning bodybuilders without coaches/trainers tend to exercise the muscles that they can see and spend most of their exercise time doing isolation exercises requiring them to lift objects in front of their bodies. As a result, the anterior muscles become proportionally stronger than the posterior ones. The first result of this imbalance in exercise programming is a new habitually poor posture, generally seen as a hunching forward with rounded shoulders. This posture limits range of motion and provides another unwanted consequence during sport, exercise, and work: a posterior weakness-driven shoulder pain. What is occurring here is that the posterior musculature is not strong enough to counter even the low level of postural muscle tension produced by the newly stronger anterior musculature. Further, the posterior musculature cannot generate enough force during stretching exercise to pull the anterior muscles through their entire range of motion. It will become a vicious downward cycle unless corrective programming is initiated. Corrective programming does not encompass prescription of isolation exercises; it is the implementation of a program utilizing large scale exercises that are resisted in multiple axes.

While there is essentially no risk of decreased range of motion or performance with proper yoga training, improper programming of yoga exercises could ultimately result in negative adaptations in mobility. If the exercises included in the program of exercise are not performed correctly or a balance of anterior and posterior, lateral and medial, and superior and inferior work is not included, there is a risk of loss of mobility. Learning and performing correct yoga posture techniques is essential to the improvement of mobility. Constructing correct yoga sequences to include in training is just as critical.

A GENERIC DESCRIPTION OF A YOGA POSTURE

There is a process common to all yoga postures. The correct procedure is to use the bodyweight and an agonist muscle or muscle group to move a body segment in order to develop slight tension in a target antagonist muscle, muscle group, or muscle groups. As the end of the possible range of motion is reached, the position is held until the perception of muscle tension fades. This will occur at about ten seconds into the posture hold and marks the point of release for beginners. For more advanced trainees, when the perception of stretch reduces at about ten seconds, a second gentle advance along the joint's range of motion is attempted and held for up to another 20 seconds. Throughout the performance of any posture, there should be a concerted effort to relax the antagonist muscles so they will yield to the pull of the agonists. By learning how to relax an antagonist muscle you can move more deeply into the range of motion and enhance movement capacity; this way, a more acute angle between two body segments is achieved. This process yields progressively greater range of motion over time. A key concept for this process is to be slow and gentle; if too much tension is developed too quickly, the safeguard reflexes within the nervous system will be activated. It is fairly simple to assess the execution of correct yoga position. If there is pain, uncontrolled muscle shaking, and/or an involuntary contraction of antagonist muscle, you are doing it wrong. Back off on the distance into the range of motion attempted, let the engaged muscles (antagonists) relax, and then proceed more carefully during the next repetition or in the next session.

While it is becoming much more common to see athletes participating in yoga to improve sport-specific range of motion, its cousin, stretching, has become a bit of a taboo for pre-exercise and pre-competition preparation. The reason for this: there can be short-lived performance decrements following static stretching (8, 9), although research results have been equivocal (10). One of these negative effects is potentially inhibited muscle activation, something needed during many multi-joint exercises and during any movement that requires the expression of agility. It is much more appropriate to include dynamic flexibility exercises at the beginning of the training session, especially prior to any high intensity conditioning activities.

BALANCE AND COORDINATION

Another of the benefits of yoga training is the improvement or enhancement of balance and movement coordination.

The foundations of balance and coordination are formed by processing sensory information and then synchronizing muscular contractions in order to adjust and stabilize body position. Although they are independent motor abilities, balance and coordination are closely related due to their reliance on the sensorimotor system; they both rely on visual, vestibular (inner ear), and proprioceptive (your sense of your body's position in space) inputs. Sensory feedback plays an important role in the control of movement. To greatly simplify a complex system, the sensorimotor system is organized so that information from the periphery (anything not the brain) is related to the brain or spinal cord and processed there. The resulting motor output (movement) is guided by further sensory input as it occurs.

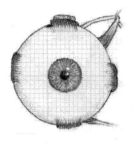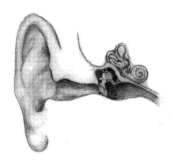

Figure 3-7. The basic anatomical tools of balance and coordination are the eye and the inner ear which provide a great deal of sensory and environmental input to the brain.

Balance is generally defined as the ability to maintain the body's center of gravity within its base of support (the mass of the body supported over whatever parts of the body are touching the ground) and can be categorized as either static balance or dynamic balance.

Static balance is the ability to maintain the body in static equilibrium. There is a distribution of body mass so that there is no movement. All of the body's mass is spread equally around a central point. Standing yoga poses are examples of static balance.

Dynamic balance brings something new to the table and requires the body to maintain equilibrium during movement. When one is walking there is a forward-directed disequilibrium. The center of the mass of the body is not over its base of support at times during the stride and the resulting unbalanced force drives movement. However, the body does not fall down. It maintains a dynamic balance, meaning that the movement is effectively controlled.

Both static and dynamic balance requires effective multi-system integration in order to control body position. An interruption, interference, or deficit in any part of the sensorimotor system can result in a loss of balance. The most innocuous result of a loss of balance is a stumble or bobble; a more severe result is injury.

Balance exerts a powerful effect on exercise technique. Poor balance is associated with reducing exercise efficiency and performance. Poor balance during exercise movements is also associated with falls or injury. Improving balance, specific to the desired exercise, is a critical component of training. Accuracy of motion and balance, the latter resulting from the former, are best developed through repetitive execution of the intended movement WITH ACCOMPANYING INSTRUCTION. A trainee cannot see his body in a pose or see himself in motion. An external pair of eyes can help provide feedback so the trainee can begin associating a kinesthetic sensation with effective posture and movement.

Balance training, performing specialized exercises on unstable surfaces, has recently grown in popularity in sport and professional fitness practice. Although balance training has proved valuable in rehabilitation settings, specifically in regards to functional ankle instability, there is virtually no compelling evidence that suggests the inclusion of training on unstable surfaces has any real and tangible effect on overall fitness. In fact, recent thesis data has demonstrated that instability training added to normal training did not enhance any element of fitness or performance (12). Nonetheless, with the aid of the media many equipment companies and fitness professionals have capitalized on this trend by promoting "balance" training (on unstable surfaces) as a crucial component of most fitness programs. Balance training implements such as stability balls (shouldn't they be called instability balls?), wobble boards, foam pads, and balance discs, all share a common purpose. They eliminate the trainee's stable contact with solid ground. As an aside, shoe choice is also important as improper shoes can unintentionally introduce an unstable platform. Balance training with these implements results in the body recruiting a great deal of peripheral musculature to attempt to control balance and not fall over. Proponents of these devices suggest that this will increase the effectiveness of training and produce better balance. However, a tremendously large oversight with that logic is that unstable surfaces improve the technique of whatever exercise is performed on them, exercises that are largely non-repeatable. If you cannot create reliable and repeatable movement patterns, you cannot improve technique and, worse, undesirable movement errors can be introduced.

Balance is skill specific. The majority of popular balance tools only work to improve static balance, which may not transfer to most real-world applications that require dynamic balance. Run the Stork Test (a test of static balance) on a group of athletes and a group of people and you will find very similar results between groups. However, put both groups through their paces in a sport environment and you will see that dynamic balance is quite different in favor of the athletes. Another major argument against balance training is that using implements that do not allow ground contact will ultimately reduce body control and the effectiveness of the exercise (13). Further, use of balance training implements does not allow for sufficient loading to induce strength gains which in many instances is the stated and primary purpose of training. It is worthwhile to note that the information labels on most stability ball packaging specifically advise against using them in weighted exercises or for any other purpose other than bodyweight support (as in stretching). There have been several high profile collegiate and professional athletes who have ended their seasons prematurely when the ball they were doing weighted exercises on popped from overload and induced ligament tears and fractures.

Considering all of the above, yoga training is a safer and more effective balance training system than the modern novelties that are so commonly marketed.

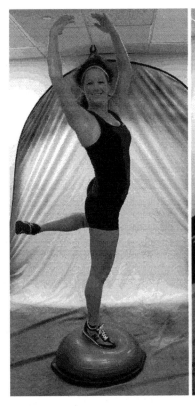 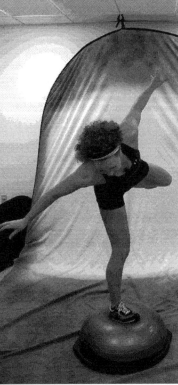

Figure 3-8. Balance on an unstable structure is difficult even for the most trained and graceful. Even if it is potentially difficult, the use of unstable work in a training program may not cross over and improve balance in a stable environment.

Coordination is a vital piece of the agility puzzle. When innately present or developed through practice, effective coordination allows a trainee to learn body movements and larger scale movement patterns and to perform them efficiently, effectively, and reliably. Simply put, coordination is the ability to synchronize and order muscle activities so an intended movement can be performed without error. Coordination affects strength in two ways. First, it allows the muscles to fire in an efficient order to maximize force production. Second, it affects performance through the precise timing of force production during a movement. These are the primary mechanisms of how yoga benefits strength over the first few months of training.

A lack of coordination is evident to virtually anyone who pays close attention while watching someone during any movement, be it lifting, running, swimming, anything. If the trainee moves in an unsynchronized manner (uncoordinated), there will be uneven flexion and extension of joints during a bilateral movement, erratic movement velocities, odd balance asymmetries, and a general lack of ease in performance.

The process of learning a new movement, all the way through coordinated proficiency, occurs through sequential learning in which one part of a task is learned before the next. Although the process of learning is sequential, it is a quite variable process between individuals. The basic teaching/learning premise is simple. It has four steps:

1. Briefly explain the movement ... or listen to the explanation,
2. Demonstrate how to do it ... or watch carefully,
3. Let them do it ... or give it a try,
4. Give feedback and repeat *ad nauseum* ... or listen to corrections and try again.

The best results come with practice of the new exercise while focusing on proper technique. Proper technique and coordination is not developed through mindless repetitions of partial movements or waving the arms and legs about in the air approximating technique. You didn't learn to drive a car by pretending. We don't learn to exercise that way either. Positive learning only occurs when the exercise environment is similar, in terms of loading, performance, tempo, and structure, to the intended movement.

FATIGUE

There is one final aspect of coordination that we need to consider. When we train, we get tired. If we train hard enough to induce fitness gain, fatigue is inevitable. Muscular fatigue impairs coordination (14) and we all have experienced this in some manner. This plays into the timing of training intended to improve balance and coordination. Although we strive to move in a coordinated manner in every exercise movement we do, there will be times later in our workouts where coordination will be dulled. In the untrained through intermediate trainees, this means that the best time for including exercises requiring high amounts of balance and coordination, or if learning a new exercise, is at the beginning of the workout. This ensures that the neuromuscular system is fresh and has the best chance for rapidly connecting the neural dots of good technique and avoids the deleterious effects of fatigue. In yoga, more demanding postures may need to be inserted later in the session. In order to ensure coordination is ready for such, a lower stress posture should be inserted just prior to the more demanding pose in order to dissipate the effects of fatigue on coordination. Recovery is essential to progress and this extends to adaptations that promote good coordination.

ENDURANCE

Let's consider endurance as a single entity for a moment. Endurance is primarily a bioenergetic phenomenon that describes the ability to deliver both oxygen and energetic nutrients to the working muscles at adequate rates and for a long enough duration to accomplish the task at hand. In this case, that involves holding a single yoga posture or completing a complete session of training.

Keep in mind, endurance is not just important for doing exercise, it is important for keeping us alive. Any number of research studies have produced a correlation between lower cardiorespiratory fitness (endurance) and higher death rates from cardiorespiratory disease, cancer, and in several papers, all-cause mortality (15, 16, 17).

We do have to note that these are correlational papers and do not establish causality. The papers almost always suggest that condition A is present at the same time as condition B, not that A causes B. Regardless, it has been well established that those with the lowest degree of endurance are likely at the highest risk of mortality. We can loosely suggest that those in the lowest 25% of the population are at the greatest risk. There is a fairly significant reduction in deaths in the next higher 25% in fitness and this is where the practice of yoga can make a great contribution. In the top 50% of fitness, the death rate does not drop much at all compared to the transition from untrained to yoga trained (this does not imply yoga is superior to other exercise systems, just that it is effective in this application with this population).

If we are doing yoga training, there are numerous periods of muscular contraction which can only be sustained by delivery of energy to the muscle. In this type of endurance, the storage, delivery, and break down of glycogen (chains of glucose), glucose, and fat is of primary concern. These metabolic processes are the limiters and facilitators of performance. When we run out, we have to slow way down in order to use the next available source of energy, protein. Using protein as an energy source is a very slow process and not very efficient. If you've ever seen a marathoner or ultra-distance runner crawl across the finish line, it's primarily because they have run out of readily available carbohydrate and fat and have switched to protein as an energy source. This is different than "hitting the wall" or "bonking" during a distance race. That occurs simply because the runner has adopted a race pace that requires energy at a rate that his aerobic capacity cannot deliver. At some point he will have to slow to a much slower pace where efficient aerobic function, and hopefully recovery, can occur and allow for completion of the race. There is a gray area between outstripping the metabolic ability of the body and the total depletion of normally available energy sources, as there many variations of how each can occur. However, they both lead to the same result: slowing down or stopping.

It is unlikely that in yoga there will ever be a condition where the carbohydrate energetic substrates are depleted enough to push metabolism into utilization of protein.

That means that it is only the rate of energy supply that will affect performance of postures and successful completion of yoga training sessions.

The other component of powering yoga is the derivation of energy from fat. Fat is a very energy-rich metabolic resource with more than twice the amount of useable energy of one gram of carbohydrate. Although fat is a very energy-dense substance, it takes a lot of time to break it down from its triglyceride form in your fat cells into more accessible fatty acids. Furthermore, this is only the first step in the process. Next, the body must move those fatty acids to the blood, then into the cell, then further break them down, move them into the mitochondria, then finally utilize their available energy. One can access fat even by starting very slowly, from sitting still up to a moderately paced jog (18). It is on this level of the metabolic expenditure continuum that yoga sits. A benefit of yoga training is that it does enhance one's ability to break down and deliver fatty acids in support of other endurance activity. Enhancement of the body's ability to mobilize and use fat to power exercise is a primary adaptation related to continuous endurance.

ARE YOU MOBILE?

There is any number of range-of-motion assessments available for use. In fact, there are entire textbooks, many of them, that describe various tests for range of motion around virtually every joint in the body. These quantitative tests are quite useful in a clinical rehabilitation environment, but in fitness practice it is more common to use qualitative assessments such as simply evaluating the ability of a trainee to assume a correct exercise position and move through the complete associated range of motion. This latter type of assessment requires the assessor to be cognizant of the anatomical reference points for the start and end points of the relevant range of motion. This is a limitation of such assessments, as most coaches and trainers have not thought of or been taught exercise technique with consideration of anatomical determinants of range of motion. In the exercise description presented later, specific anatomical segment associations have been described to ensure that each exercise can be objectively evaluated for completeness of range of motion. To address the issue of mobility posed above, if you can perform the exercises as described, achieving the complete range of motion, then you are mobile.

REFERENCES

1. Fabre, J., et al. Age-related deterioration in flexibility is associated with health-related quality of life in nonagenarians. Journal of Geriatric Physical Therapy. 2007. 30(1):16–22.

2. Buchman, A.S., et al. Physical activity and motor decline in older persons. Muscle & Nerve. 2007. 35(3): 354–362.

3. US Department of Health and Human Services. Health, United States, 2010: With Special Feature on Death and Dying. DHHS Publication No. 2011-1232, Washington, DC, 2011.

4. Wells, G.D., M. Elmi, and S. Thomas. Physiological correlates of golf performance. Journal of Strength and Conditioning Research. 2009. 23(3): 741-750.

5. Martin, S.B., et al. The rationale for the sit and reach test revisited. Measurement in Physical Education and Exercise Science. 1998. 2: 85-92.

6. Grenier, S.G., C. Russell, and S.M. McGill. Relationships between lumbar flexibility, sit-and-reach test, and a previous history of low back discomfort in industrial workers. Canadian Journal of Applied Physiology. 2003. 28: 165-177.

7. Nereng, A, JP Porcari, C Camic, C Gillette and C Foster. Hot Yoga: Go Ahead and Turn Up the Heat. ACE Certified News 1-2, 2013. https://www.acefitness.org/certifiednews/images/article/pdfs/YogaStudy.pdf

8. Behm, D.G., D.C. Button, and J.C. Butt. Factors affecting force loss with prolonged stretching. Canadian Journal of Applied Physiology. 2001. 26(3):261-272.

9. Fowles, J.R., D.G. Sale, and J.D. MacDougall. Reduced strength after passive stretch of the human plantar flexors. Journal of Applied Physiology. 2000. 89(3):1179-1188.

10. Ryan, E.D., et al. Do practical durations of stretching alter muscle strength? A dose-response study. Medicine and Science in Sports and Exercise. 2008. 40(8):1529-37.

11. Sheppard, J.M. and W.B. Young. Agility literature review: classifications, training and testing. Journal of Sports Science. 2006. 24(9): 915-28.

12. Brumbalow, J. Meta-analysis of stability ball training on fitness performance. Thesis preliminary data. Midwestern State University, Wichita Falls, Texas, 2011.

13. Behm, D.G., K. Anderson, and R.S. Curnew. Muscle force and activation under stable and unstable conditions. Journal of Strength and Conditioning Research. 2002. 16: 416–422.

14. Taylor, J.L., J.E. Butler, and S.C. Gandevia. Changes in muscle afferents, motoneurons and motor drive during muscle fatigue. European Journal of Applied Physiology. 2000. 83 (2-3): 106-115.

15. Blair, S.N., et al. Changes in physical fitness and all-cause mortality: A prospective study of healthy and unhealthy men. Journal of the American Medical Association. 1995. 273:1093–1098.

16. Carnethon, M.R., M. Gulati, and P. Greenland. Prevalence and cardiovascular disease correlates of low cardiorespiratory fitness in adolescents and adults. Journal of the American Medical Association. 2005. 294:2981–2988.

17. Lee, D.C., et al. Mortality trends in the general population: the importance of cardiorespiratory fitness. Journal of Psychopharmacology. 2010. 24(4 Supplement):27-35.

18. Achten, J. and A.E. Jeukendrup. Relation between plasma lactate concentration and fat oxidation rates over a wide range of exercise intensities. International Journal of Sports Medicine. 2004. 25(1):32-37.

"When something is important enough, you do it even if the odds are not in your favor."

Elon Musk

4 – PERSONAL AND ORGANIZATIONAL PREPARATIONS FOR YOGA TRAINING

Before you actually start a yoga training session there are a few items that require attention. You don't just "do" yoga; you plan yoga sessions. You plan the place you will be doing them; you plan for your personal needs. If you are learning, you plan to find a competent teacher, and if you are teaching, you plan to be competent and prepared. Professionals do not fly by the seat of their pants, because failing to plan is planning to fail. This refers to your ability to deliver excellent instruction and to the ability of programs to efficiently deliver fitness.

A PLAN

A yoga training session has a purpose. It is not an assortment of randomly selected and randomly ordered exercise postures. A competent yoga trainer should match the session to the intent of a longer term training goal. Each session should be choreographed in advance, should include exercises that flow or link together in sequence fluidly, and should be adaptable for the varied levels of student capability present. For a healthy beginning trainee who intends to improve basic range of motion and fitness, the characteristics of a good yoga session are:

1. A proper and efficient warm up—this is accomplished through a progressive series of postures.
2. Attention to detail of where to place hands and feet on the mat and where the body should be upon the mat—you wouldn't start a forward lunging movement standing on the front of the mat or facing to the side.
3. The intent of the session should be clearly understood by the instructor, communicated to the trainees, and reflected in the choices and sequence of exercise postures included.

4. Instruction and teaching points should be worded such that they are appropriate to the range of ability levels of students in the class—this means that the instructions and cues used by an instructor will be repeated in varied forms so beginners and advanced trainees alike can understand them.

5. Instruction on breath control—when to breathe as one moves through the postures—should be clearly communicated.

6. Demonstrations should be visible to all present.

7. Students should feel comfortable and not be overwhelmed by new expectations—yoga tends to be best conducted in a relaxed atmosphere.

A PLACE

While yoga training can be done virtually anywhere, there are a few considerations required before getting into a session. What makes a room acceptable? There are some things that apply more to teaching environments than to home based practice, but the basics are just that: basic needs for effective practice.

1. As a warm muscle is more extensible than a cold one, a moderately warm room is quite beneficial. A comfortable ambient temperature allows the student to focus less on thermal comfort and more on performing exercises. Hot environments are not necessary as the body in motion will create heat quickly (it has also been demonstrated that while hot rooms get students warmed-up more quickly, the long term results from yoga done in a hot room and yoga in a comfortable room are the same). On the opposite end of the spectrum, it is rather uncomfortable and progress comes more slowly when practicing yoga in cold, air conditioned spaces.

2. The exercise floor should ideally be wood. Smooth and level surfaces are needed so the yoga mat sits evenly on the surface for trainee comfort in sitting and lying

poses. The smooth hard surface is best for providing contact and friction between the mat and floor which prevents mat sliding.

3. Basic good practice means that all exercise environments should be clean. Although trainees will exercise on their own personal mats, they will have their face near the floor and their personal effects on the floor. A dirty floor is off-putting and will not inspire confidence and return business. Keep the floor clean and swept.

4. There must be enough space to move through all planned exercise postures. While it is normal for trainees in yoga studio practices to practice in close proximity, personal space must be attended to, as cramped trainees will be limited in both their focus and their ability to achieve complete range of motion.

5. Home-based practice can be done in any adequately open space. For commercial practices an empty room is ideal. This means that the room should be devoid of furniture. Mirrors can be strategically placed such that trainees can see themselves and the instructor so they can model their movements based on what they see. Mirrors can be a help or a distraction. They may cause students to look at themselves or others in the mirror rather than focusing on their own kinesthetic awareness and execution of the postures being learned. As such they may or may not be present in a studio.

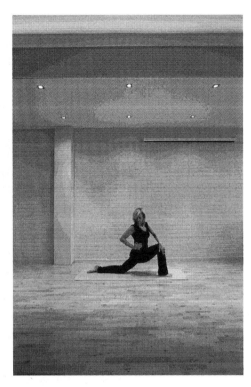

Figure 4-1. A typical yoga studio.

Yoga is an infinitely transportable exercise system. You will never be at a loss for a space to practice. Be it a smooth patch of ground outside, the floor of a bathroom, kitchen, or any room of the house with enough floor space, the deck of a boat (as long as it's bigger than a bass boat or dinghy), basketball court, dojo mat, office floor, you get the idea. Your ability to practice goes with you everywhere. This can be important, as regular participation in exercise is what all fitness professionals desire for their clients. It's what medical professionals recommend. It's what brings about the best fitness improvements.

A MAT

One of the most identifiable pieces of personal equipment associated with the practice of yoga is the yoga mat. Every gym will require you to have one (or in some instances you can rent one) in order to be allowed to practice. The mat has a few specific functions in the gym. First, it defines "your space" on the yoga studio floor. Second, the cushioning it provides (it's just a small bit) makes working on the usual hard surfaces of the yoga studio or gym tolerable. And finally, the mat acts as a tool that helps the hands and feet stay in place on the mat and the mat stay in place on the floor, both combining to create a good foundation on which to move.

Choosing a "yoga" mat is important. When buying a mat, you need to make sure it is a good quality one. It is best if you have seen the mat and felt its surface and cushion. Ask other trainees and instructors for opinions and advice on the best products, especially if you plan on buying the mat from an online merchant. There are a wide selection of thicknesses, prices, and colors available but there are some basic things to look for:

1. The mat needs to have a sticky surface. Most yoga mats have this as a normal feature in the form of a rubbery outer coating (over an inner foam cushion). While they may look similar, camping mats do not have the same degree of cushion nor the non-slip outer coating. Similarly don't choose the thicker Pilates mat, while they are more padded, they too lack the non-slip coating on the underside. The lack of the non-slip characteristic in these two similar looking mats makes performing yoga exercises less effective and occasionally can make them more dangerous.

2. The non-slip rubber coating present on yoga mats can be different between manufacturers. Inspect the labels carefully and feel the tack of the coating. Cheaper PVC (poly-vinyl-chloride) derived coatings will generally not be durable

enough for long term use and will lack the traction to keep the mat in place during use. It is a much better option to purchase latex rubber or composites to provide the best durability and traction. In terms of thickness, there again are numerous thicknesses. The best choices are 3/16" or 1/4" thick. Too thin of a mat limits cushioning. Thin mats can deform during use and too thick of a mat can interfere with posture stability and motor control.

3. Yoga mats need to be prepared for first use and maintained for continued use. When you buy a new mat and run your fingers across the surface, it will feel oily. As part of the manufacturing and shipping process they are treated with light oil. The oil prevents mats from fusing to each other during manufacture and to itself after it's rolled and packaged for sale. To ensure that the mat provides friction to the floor and to your feet, clean the mat prior to first use by using soapy warm water and a damp cloth. Then wipe all residual moisture off with a dry cloth. You will sweat during yoga training and the sweat will end up on the mat. It is good practice to wipe down your mat routinely to ensure you are exercising on a sanitary surface. The sweat-sanitize cycle can help cultivate the ideal sticky surface for your mat. This also points out a very good reason to own your own mat. If you rent or borrow, you are sharing sweat with others.

Instructors should have a few back-up mats on hand. Some trainee will invariably forget theirs and need a loaner. It is typical that new students will turn up with brand new mats (and the oil treatment has not been removed from the mat's surface) and sweaty palms (they are nervous in an environment new to them). They will slip around on the oily surface, have difficulty maintaining stability, and they will look around and notice that no one else appears to be having the same problem. An observant yoga teacher will have a seasoned mat they can quickly put on the top of the new mat to make the student better able to perform AND to make them feel a little less self-conscious. After the session the instructor should then explain the perils of new mats and how to correct the slippage problem.

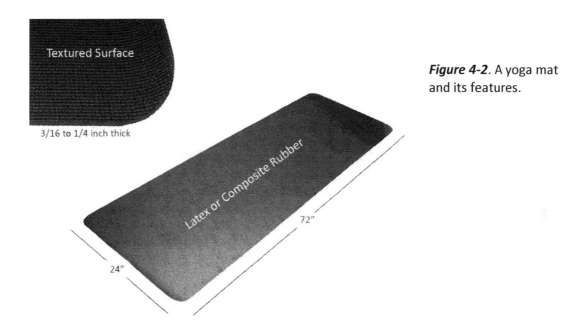

Figure 4-2. A yoga mat and its features.

A final, and quite personal, aspect of choosing a yoga mat is what it looks like. You can choose a color based on personal favorite or simple whim. However, the colors in an environment can affect individual mood state positively or negatively. In general people tend to choose brighter colors as motivational. Whatever color and/or decorative design you choose, get a "good" one and make it individual for easy recognition ... and then like Linus and his blanket, you will get quite attached to your yoga mat.

OTHER PERSONAL ITEMS

There are a number of other items that can make the yoga training session more effective and more comfortable. Some are dubbed as essential and some are simply useful.

A TOWEL

A towel is an essential tool of all exercise training, indoor and out.

> "A towel ... is about the most massively useful thing an interstellar hitchhiker can have. Partly it has great practical value - you can wrap it around you for warmth ... you can wave your towel in emergencies as a distress signal, and of course dry yourself off with it if it still seems to be clean enough."
>
> *Douglas Adams*
> Hitchhiker's Guide to the Galaxy

Every hard-core weightlifter and powerlifter has a towel in their gym bag. They can be found in martial arts dojos and boxing gyms. They are a ubiquitous element of personal exercise equipment. In a yoga session, a towel is extremely handy to have with you. Sweat on the yoga mat reduces the friction between the foot and mat, making stability and balance more difficult. Sweaty hands can create support issues between hand and mat and can create posture hold problems if the hand-grip slides due to wetness. A towel can be used to eliminate mat or body moisture problems in transition times between postures.

Everyone sweats. Some people more than others. If you tend to sweat a lot or don't like the sensation of sweat running down your skin, a towel is essential. The towel should be kept neatly at the side or front of the mat. While a huge bath towel is not needed, there are relatively large specific-to-yoga mat towels (they have sticky pads on one side so they don't slide away). For many trainees, a smaller hand towel will do nicely. The only real criteria for towel choice are that it be clean and absorbent.

BLOCKS

Not everyone in a yoga session has all of the required range of motion or anatomical body segment lengths that enable assuming an exercise posture unaided. A good yoga teacher or studio should have blocks and other props that will aid trainees in assuming correct final postures, or that will aid them in moving towards acquiring the ability to do so over time. A yoga block is simply a piece of high density plastic/rubber that is used as an extension of the arm if the trainee cannot reach the floor. Its function is to allow the student to "touch" the floor as an aid to balance or to help provide something to push against the floor to help attain anatomical alignments in certain poses. The block looks a lot like a brick, with some being 50 mm (2 inches) thick or 25 mm (1 inch) thick. The thinner versions are sometimes preferable to the thicker as they are lighter, easier to move, and slightly more comfortable to sit on (during periods of verbal instruction).

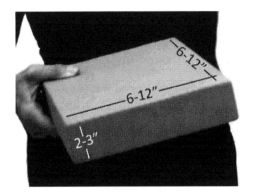

Figure 4-3. Yoga blocks.

A STRAP

There are instances where we need to be able to pull against the feet or to join the hands behind the back to assume a correct position. Range of motion insufficiency or particularly short anatomical body segments may prohibit some individuals from doing some postures or making progress towards performing them appropriately. A short (less than one yard or meter) canvas or other robust fabric strap (like the material from which luggage straps are made) allow the two body segments (hand-foot or hand-hand) to be indirectly connected. This enables appropriate force to be generated that pulls or twists the body or body part into appropriate anatomical alignment.

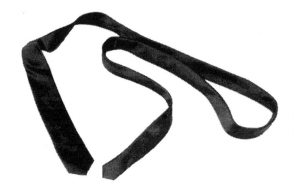

Figure 4-4. A strap can be used by those with limited mobility during postures such as the seated forward fold and a closed sage twist. A simple dress tie can be quite an economical strap.

CLOTHING

Any clothing worn to a yoga training session must allow unrestricted movement and it should conform to the shape or form of the body. This does not mean, as many people immediately assume, spandex or high price trendy workout clothes. Clothing must simply be comfortable, stretchable, and breathable. Even old school grey sweats will work. T-shirts and stretchy shorts work just fine too. Whatever is worn needs to allow full range of motion movement for the trainee and allow the instructor to see anatomical alignments. The former provides the best individual performance; the latter affords the best opportunity for teaching.

Figure 4-5. Clothing appropriate for yoga.

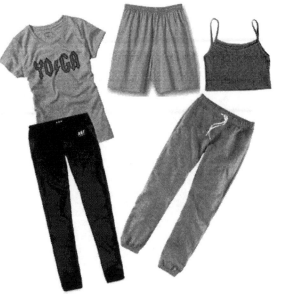

The original Olympians trained and competed in the buff. The best cooling of the body is provided by direct exposure of the skin to the environment. Less clothing also provides the least restriction to movement, so there is somewhat of a basis for wearing limited clothing during training, as permitted by environmental conditions. Also, when people get fit, they like to wear less to show off their hard-won fitness gains. It's good to be confident and proud of your gains but certain activities require certain apparel considerations.

In any facility used by multiple people, especially where there is contact of skin to shared surfaces, clothing choice is important. For group health, a barrier between the skin and contact surfaces, whether machine or floor, are needed to diminish the risk of bacterial infection spread among users (reviewed in 1). Staphylococcus from one person's skin to shared surface contact can infect many other people who put their skin on the same surface. This can be easily solved by repetitive cleaning of contact surfaces throughout the day, but it's generally easier for all involved to just wear clothes that stop skin-to-surface contact. This is as easy as simply wearing shirts for men, rather than going shirtless, and wearing minimal tops for women to effectively attenuate the spread of disease.

Another aspect of bacteria and clothing is related to how the fabric of the clothes you choose to wear affects your own personal aromatic presence (aka, stink factor). A recent study demonstrated very nicely that cotton exercise clothing does a better job at preventing post exercise bacterial growth than clothing made of polyester materials (2). This has a direct impact on everyone around you if you should wear the same workout clothing in sequential sessions. You might be able to get away with it with cotton clothing, but why not just wash your gear between sessions? It lowers disease risk AND your training peers will thank you.

Yoga training is conducted in bare feet. Shoes are, by custom—similar to martial arts facilities—left at the door, in the locker room, or, at worst, to the side of the exercise floor. Street shoes carry dirt and contamination onto the exercise floor and this is not acceptable in terms of customer satisfaction or health.

Other than the issues of clothes and shoes, everything else about yoga apparel is wide open. Slave to fashion or minimalist couture is unimportant; it's the training that is important. Cheryl Tiegs once proclaimed that "It's very important to have the right clothing to exercise in. If you throw on an old T-shirt or sweats, it's not inspiring for your workout." We'd like to think that the results of training are what is inspiring, but if cool gear gets you to the session on time, every time, that works too.

YOGA SESSION STUDENT ETIQUETTE

What is expected in terms of student behavior? Each yoga practice will have a specific set of guidelines for student conduct. A copy will generally be given to the student at the sign-up time for classes. Alternatively, most yoga practices with an internet presence will also have these guidelines available online.

All group exercise environments must be structured so that instructor-student interactions can occur effectively. This means that there is always a noise restriction in place, either formally or informally; the students have to be able to hear what the instructor is saying. In some instances, such as in dance based exercise systems like Zumba, the instructor has to use a microphone and PA to deliver instruction. This is not the case in yoga where the environment is usually a much more peaceful and sedate space. As yoga practice requires individual focus on personal learning, movement, and body position, individual and group behavior should reflect that need. This means that when it is time for the training session to begin, keep your voice down if you speak to those around you and do not compete with the instructor's voice. Some yoga studios require more silence than others, so make sure you are familiar with the rules and practices of the studio in which you are training. When in doubt, quiet is always a good idea, especially if you are waiting for a preceding class to finish up.

Group exercise is a community building activity. As such, if a number of clients have been coming and training together for many years and have built a strong community spirit, it will be common for them to have a group personality and greet each other with boisterous tales of the weekend or current life-events. This sense of belonging and community is precisely what is desired as it promotes long term exercise habits and client satisfaction; however, a gentle reminder is sometimes needed to get the group focused on their exercises and mindful of the fact that they have gotten to where they are by focused practice in a quiet environment.

As a student, it is important to listen to instructions carefully and to look at the instructor for any physical cues provided through demonstration. If you are new, don't set up your mat in the back, the instructor is in front and they are there to help you. They can't do that if they can't see you way back in the back corner.

Try to stay with the sequence of teaching. Being in perfect synchrony with others around you (who may be more experienced than you) is not useful, or even desired. Yoga is individualized and as a beginner you are working towards getting into the correct position in the allocated time, not towards immediately moving into perfect posture and holding it for exactly so many seconds or so many breaths. If you have just gotten your body into a good semblance of the posture when it's time to move to the next, or even if you didn't, that's just fine. Move to the next posture of instruction. You're learning. Learning proper position is exquisitely important, so don't stress or get frustrated. Even if you do get a little frustrated, don't just do your own thing. If the instructor sees you having difficulty they will give you cues or adapt the posture to aid you. It is a rare occasion that an instructor will give someone leave to freestyle as that creates a somewhat confusing environment for the group as a whole.

You can unilaterally choose to modify what you are doing if you are in pain or feel what is being asked of you is well beyond your ability. You are a client receiving a service and a good yoga instructor should be able to observe and teach modifications for every exercise posture they use. Individualization and adaptation for the client is part of the job and under no circumstances should the client be made to feel inferior or victimized by needing accommodation.

THE FIRST DAY

Going along to a yoga class for the first time can be quite a daunting experience, especially if the trainee is coming in alone and knows no one in the group. The student should ensure that they introduce themselves to the instructor and flag up that they are new with no idea of what to expect and how to proceed (be honest!). The instructor should take note and ensure that the student is well placed to hear and see instruction.

Before a yoga session starts, a beginner will see a bunch of what they perceive as competent trainees doing lots of different pre-session rituals. The beginner, based on this observation, will think they are not doing something they should be doing. Uncertainty and a feeling of inadequacy will start creeping in. If no one tells a beginner precisely what to do and when to do it, the door is open for dissatisfaction and dropping out. If a yoga instructor is trying to sell a service, having the first experience a student has be one of inattention is not good business practice. Every instructor and every advanced trainee was once a beginner and should make every effort to aid newbies in their initial sessions: the instructor because their business depends on satisfaction and return clientele, the other trainees because the community needs to be positive to grow.

WHAT WOULD MAKE A TRAINEE A PERFECT TRAINEE?

There really is no "perfect" trainee but there are a number of characteristics of successful trainees:

1. Someone who listens to instructions and who is mindful of developing their own personal abilities. Yoga instructors constantly observe students and use a variety of techniques, verbal and physical, to teach modification of postures. Listen and watch for teaching instructions relative to adapting a posture. Sometimes you may not be sure if the comment is directed to you, so you should proactively try the adaptation. If your body feels any different or more at ease having carried out the instruction, it was meant for you.

2. Someone who displays proper self-focus, i.e., does not look around the room at how everyone else is doing and maintains their mat and physical presence within their own space.

3. Someone who lets the instructor do their job and does not offer correction to other students.

4. Someone who is at ease, comfortable, and focused on the task at hand, which in this case is the relatively tall task of bending, twisting, and holding your body in positions that develop your ability to move through a complete range of motion and develop you into a more fit individual. Unfortunately, this status generally comes only after years of progressive yoga practice.

WHAT NOT TO DO

The overall key is to not interfere with other trainees such that they are prevented from being in a position to learn and refine postures and skills during training. There are some specific issues that might be considered egregious errors:

1. Wearing shoes in class: A problem with sanitation and tradition.
2. Entering a session after it has started: Many studios won't allow late access as it is disruptive and limits your progress.
3. Leaving the session prior to completion: Disrupts others and limits your progress.
4. Taking a phone into the session: Disruptive to everyone.
5. Talking louder than the teacher: Neither you nor other students benefit from instruction if it can't be heard.
6. Chatting to the people near you during the class: Distracts you and those around you from proper focus.
7. Asking many questions during instruction: While asking for help is acceptable, asking too many questions during class disrupts the flow of the class and can prevent the training effect from being delivered to all students in the session. Save questions for after the session ends when student-instructor dialogue won't interfere with the conduct of the session.

Some yoga practices cultivate a sense of attention to the Indian roots of yoga through adoption of specific Sanskrit greetings, chants, and other eastern ritual elements. If the class contains some or all of these elements, you need not feel compelled to join in; if you prefer, just stay quiet, bow your head slightly, and wait for the others to finish and proceed to the actual training session.

WHAT DO YOU LOOK FOR IN A GOOD YOGA INSTRUCTOR?

Not all teachers are the same, in any field. Some can be quite conversational, some a little dictatorial; some are encyclopedic, casual, inclusive; some are a little of everything. A good yoga instructor will generally do the following as part of a class:

1. Greet students before class in a friendly manner. This should enable them to identify new trainees and welcome regulars.

2. Determine if anyone has any injury or other limitation that would affect one's health or ability to participate in the session. This should happen before the start of the session.

3. Help beginners find a space in the studio and manage others in spacing themselves. It is much easier as a beginner to be nearer the teacher so you can clearly see and hear instructions.

4. Move through the studio space when possible to make corrections or modify position. The instructor has a responsibility to ensure that everyone is responding to the exercises in an appropriate and safe manner. Moving to and helping those trainees who are a little behind or who are having difficulty is important as it facilitates the entire class in performing the same exercise, or adaptation thereof, at roughly the same time.

5. Ask students how they are feeling to ensure their bodies accommodated the stress placed upon them successfully, and will offer help with practical issues or any practice related questions.

CHARACTERISTICS OF A GOOD YOGA TEACHER

1. A good self-practice. Yoga is a large set of learned skills and the instructor needs to continually develop their own abilities in practice and teaching.

2. A welcoming attitude. New students should feel part of the group from the first visit and veterans should feel at home. Students should not feel frustrated by the experience in any way … other than that which normally accompanies learning and trying to master new skills.

3. A sense of humor in an instructor makes learning and the learning environment less intimidating.

4. A keen eye for detail. The instructor must be able to see what the trainee is doing right and wrong and make appropriate commentary or instruction for the students' benefit based on those observations. Such a teacher will actively observe students from various angles and use the observations as teaching points.

5. An ability to use their voice as a tool. Good instructors vary the pitch, tone and volume of their voice during instruction. Monotone is neither calming nor exciting to listen to for any period of time.

6. A sense of duty to students. Whether presented with a beginner or a veteran student, a good instructor will adapt their practice to accommodate them. They realize that one size does not fit all. They care about the progress of every client.

Finding the right yoga teacher is a very personal thing, when you find the right one for you, you know it. There is no sure-fire way to determine if a newly minted instructor will be a great one as they are just beginning and developing their teaching acumen. One thing that is certain is that they will be motivated to try. Similarly, there is no sure-fire way to know if an experienced instructor will be the one for you. They have developed their approach to teaching over time and their adopted methods may not be precisely right for you. In both instances, the only way to tell for sure is to audition them. Almost all yoga studios offer single session or very short term packages for new potential members. All new customers should take advantage of these in order to find the best fit.

REFERENCES

1. Cohen, P.R. The skin in the gym: a comprehensive review of the cutaneous manifestations of community-acquired methicillin-resistant Staphylococcus aureus infection in athletes. Clinical Dermatology. 2008. 26(1):16-26.

2. Callewaert C, De Maeseneire E, Kerckhof FM, Verliefde A, de Wiele TV, Boon N. Microbial odor profile of polyester and cotton clothes after a fitness session. Applied Environmental Microbiology. 2014. doi: 10.1128/AEM.01422-14.

   http://aem.asm.org/content/early/2014/08/12/AEM.01422-14.long

"No problem is too small or too trivial if we can really do something about it."

Richard Feynman

5 – THE ELEMENTS OF A YOGA TRAINING SESSION

When you are training in Yoga, regardless of who the instructor is, you will see some physical and choreographic essentials consistently present in every session or workout. When a training session is constructed correctly, the trainee will perceive what seems to be a seamless series of postures and movements that transition in a logical manner. Each movement and posture should feel like a logical step in the context of moving from the previous posture into the subsequent posture. Each training session should be constructed to accomplish this "flow."

A flow, at its simplest, is a connected series of exercises that accomplishes a number of physiological goals. When properly planned and executed, a flow should:

1. Accomplish a thorough warm-up of all parts of the body to be trained.
2. Provide a level of effort or exertion high enough to provide a muscular or metabolic effect (i.e., improve fitness).
3. Provide a cool-down to ensure that all trainees have tolerated the work without health consequence.

A flow, correctly designed and delivered, also provides some mental stimuli that help develop some useful psychological outcomes.

1. The early section of the flow ramps the intensity and effort up gradually to ensure trainees have the confidence and self-efficacy to engage in the training session completely.
2. The main body of the session, where the exercises included are hardest, helps improve pain tolerance, attention, and focus.
3. The later section of the flow where the intensity/effort diminishes to the point of complete rest provides an exceptional and beneficial perception of relaxation.

From a mathematic standpoint, you might consider a flow to be a simple bell shaped curve with the effort, posture difficulty, or intensity following a normal distribution (figure 5-1). Think about this curve and the relationships it represents as you participate as a student in any yoga class. You should be able to attach the activities done within the session to specific segments of this curve. This distribution is characteristic of all yoga sessions intended for beginners through intermediates. Only the magnitude of difficulty changes, with beginners being programmed with easier postures and intermediates with more difficult postures. It is relevant here to talk about relative intensity or relative difficulty. A beginner can work extremely hard and generate high heart rates, rapid breathing, and lots of muscular activity even with "easy" movements and postures. Remember that they are untrained; everything is harder than what they are used to doing. Good instructors will ensure that trainees with different levels of training progression (beginner, intermediate, advanced) will be presented with postures and movements that deliver relevant physical challenge.

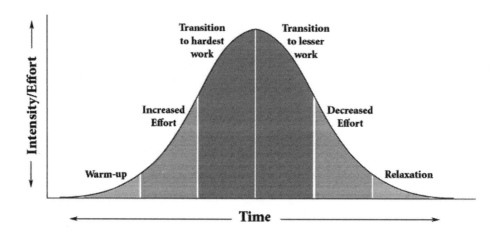

Figure 5-1. Distribution of intensity or effort associated with yoga postures over the duration of a single session.

Structure of a Warm-Up

The most obvious concept associated with creating a warm-up is that the initial movements should be executed more slowly than those occurring later in the session. Furthermore, the range of motion used at the beginning of the warm-up phase should be small. It should amplify to a full range of motion by the time more demanding postures are first included in the session. By combining attention to breath rate and overall movement in this manner, respiratory, cardiac, and skeletal muscle will have an opportunity to increase in temperature and thus maximize the effects of later exercises included in the session. It is during this phase of the training session that instructors should coach trainees to pay attention to their kinesthetic focus (where they are in space and how their body feels in various positions).

The warm-up phase begins with standing postures that progressively work on moving through the range of motion of the neck, shoulders, lumbar vertebrae, hips, knees, and ankles. Standing stretches are useful here as they are generally performed with the feet at approximately hips-width apart and the position of the body over the base of standing support aids in priming kinesthetic awareness. Use of postures with the arms overhead is important here. Full extension of the arms overhead increases the distance that blood has to travel above the heart and increases the amount of work the heart has to do to drive circulation. This all prepares the body for the upcoming more difficult exercises included in the remainder of the session.

Progression of Effort and Movements

The movements and postures included in the warm-up and transition phases of the training session are dependent on the intent of the main body of the session. Early movements should link to later postures in terms of movement pattern, joints and musculature affected, and ending stance.

For example, if a focus of a specific training session is enhancement of low back and hip range of motion, the early warm-up movements should begin as a whole body effort and then the transition elements should progressively increase in their utilization of the musculature and range of motion in those areas and reduce the focus on non-target areas.

There are some choreographic considerations made to ensure that there are smooth transitions from posture to posture. This is quite frequently dependent on how the feet are to be placed at the end of one posture and at the beginning of the subsequent posture. A well planned session will have foot placement patterns that make position changes between postures appear logical and efficient. Efficient posture changes do not require extensive time or thinking. This does not mean that every posture must follow exactly from the previous posture. In order to achieve training objectives there may be a need to change body position significantly or to provide a lower effort recovery period following a difficult posture. An intervening posture can be sandwiched between two postures in order to create a transitional base for large scale postural change or a period of lower effort.

The difficulty and effort required in the middle section of the session (where most of the training benefit will be realized) is mediated by the number and difficulty of the postures used. Postures where balance is focused on one foot or there are longer or numerous levers created (multiple joints used to maintain balance) will require more muscular exertion than postures where balance is divided more equally on both feet, and where the posture creates fewer levers. This manipulation is most directly related to "intensity" as it affects the magnitude of muscular effort needed to perform the posture. Modulating intensity is the first way to make a session more or less difficult. A second way to alter the difficulty of the session is to add more postures to the main section of the session. This relates most directly to the "volume" of training as it affects the amount of effort expended through increasing the time of exertion. Both ways of changing difficulty are viable but have slightly different purposes. The former relates to developing more strength, the latter to developing more endurance. Note that in both iterations "endurance" and range of motion are the two elements of fitness most developed. Once an individual is able to hold a posture for 15 to 30 seconds, the strength stimulus of the posture is limited.

There is a time consideration if you include more poses in the main section of a session; does the trainee have enough available time to complete the session? Most clients of a commercial yoga business will attend training two or three times per week and will do so just before work, on a lunch break, or immediately after work. This generally sets boundaries of time that cannot be breached – to do so would negatively affect the client's employment and therefore, ability to afford participation. This generally suggests that the complete training session should take no more than an hour and the number of postures that can be included in any such session are limited by time. Inclusion of strength biased postures would work well here. If, per chance, the trainee can do one or two sessions during the week and one on the weekend, a longer, endurance based session can be conducted.

Time in an individual posture is generally controlled by holding it for a specific number of breaths, convention being five breaths. Inhale for a count of three and exhale for a count of three (thus equating to about 30 seconds). To increase the amount of local muscular endurance required and developed, the count can be extended (for example, a count of five instead of three). If there is a need to increase the number of postures included in a session then the count of breath cycles can be reduced (for example, from five breaths down to three).

Cool-down and Relaxation

While the cool-down section of an exercise session achieves no direct fitness gain, it does provide a period of observation when the instructor can ensure that the trainee completed the session without medical consequence. In yoga, the cool-down is an especially important section. It creates an excellent transition into one of the key features associated with yoga practice: relaxation.

This section of the yoga session has the practitioner move from standing postures to kneeling postures, then down to seated postures, and then to a final supine posture (corpse). As the cool-down progresses, the session moves nearer to the floor and the postures reduce in the amount of exertion required until the trainee is lying effortlessly on the floor. The standard practice for duration of the final posture is five minutes. It is during this last set of transitions and the final effortless posture that the trainee will reap the positive benefits (physiological and psychological) of this facilitated relaxation. These few minutes can have a profound health benefit for the trainee so this process should never be overlooked or omitted.

"Self-education is, I firmly believe, the only kind of education there is."

Isaac Asimov

6 – ETHICS IN YOGA PRACTICE

Old School Ethics in the New World

Ethics have always been part of the world of yoga. Remember that in the Yoga Sūtras, ethics are presented as one of the eight branches:

1. Yama (ethics)
2. Niyama (discipline)
3. Asana (physical practice)
4. Pranayama (breathing)
5. Pratyahara (sensory withdrawal)
6. Dharana (concentration)
7. Dhyana (contemplation)
8. Samadhi (ecstasy)

Though we are most directly focused on the physical practices of yoga (Asana), as this is our primary area of instruction, ethics (Yama) are also brought forward into our modern practices as they can directly affect our teaching efforts.

The basic premises of yoga-based ethics are not foreign to anyone. They are similar to or part of what is considered normal ethics across many professions and cultures. Some can be considered common courtesy and apply to students as much as they do to instructors.

Do no harm – Although most commonly associated with medical practices, this ethic goes beyond not doing physical harm to your students. It also encompasses the concept of not doing harm to the confidence or the happiness of your students or associates. This ethic also extends across the realms of an instructor's personal and professional life. One should maintain integrity in work relationships and interactions with students in and out of class. The Sanskrit terms most closely aligned to this ethic are Ahimsa and Brahmacharya.

Be gracious and welcoming – This is the cornerstone of building a positive exercise experience for students. It opens the door for word-of-mouth marketing to aid in the growth of your practice. Also included here is the idea of treating all students without judgment or prejudice. The Sanskrit term most closely aligned to this ethic is Ahimsa.

Honesty is the best policy – Correctly and honestly represent yourself, what you know, and the practice of yoga in your teachings. Further, approach your professional dealings with truthfulness and respect for the other party or parties. It is also important to represent your training and scope of practice accurately. Never suggest that you can provide medical advice, or any other kind of clinical advice to anyone UNLESS you are specifically trained (professional degree in medicine, dietetics, pharmacy, etc.) to do so. If you do provide health and nutrition information or guidance, ensure that the other party clearly understands it to be YOUR opinion. The Sanskrit term most closely aligned to this ethic is Satyam.

Thou shalt not steal – While it may be tempting to do so to increase your client base. Do not attempt to recruit (poach) students by publicly or privately making negative commentary about a peer's teachings, training history, or personality. If you do your job correctly, students from ineffective or poor operations will drift towards your practice over time. The Sanskrit term most closely aligned to this ethic is Asteya.

The needs of the many outweigh the needs of the few or the one – Ensure that your teachings are benefitting the student, promoting their fitness, health, and wellbeing. This means that their needs outweigh your needs. If your classes do not meet the student's stated or obvious needs, you must not avoid altering your practice to accommodate them for the sake of your ease of delivery. If the student for some reason does not benefit from your work, you should not refrain from referring them to another instructor who may better serve their needs. You should do so without expectation of reward and without regret. Even if making them happy meant helping them find a place to fit outside your practice, don't let them leave without a positive service. The Sanskrit term most closely aligned to this ethic is Aaparigraha.

Be a life-long learner – As an exercise professional, you have an ethical duty to continue to educate yourself in the practice of Yoga. This means that your study should always be evolving. You should continue your personal studies through additional readings, seminars, workshops, and conferences. For example, we have focused on the physical aspects of yoga (Asana) and here we have an abbreviated the treatment of ethics (Yama). That leaves six other branches of yoga for you to explore over your professional life. The Sanskrit term most closely aligned to this ethic is Svadyaya.

If you're gonna talk the talk, you better walk the walk – Simply put, practice what you preach. Your integrity as an instructor can hinge on whether you actually do, or can do, the exercises and skills you are asking the trainees to perform. It also depends on your authentic belief that your practice is an example of "good practice". You must believe that the services you are providing are high quality and based in fact. The Sanskrit terms most closely aligned to this ethic are Tapas and Saucha.

Always do your best – You should always endeavor to provide the best instruction possible. You should also value and commend the success of students you teach and that of other yoga instructors when they perform well. Your attention and positive feedback to students doing well is not based on numbers; commend and praise as needed and as earned, no matter the number of students in a class. The Sanskrit term most closely aligned to this ethic is Santosha.

Humility is the foundation of all other virtues – As one becomes more skilled and successful as a professional, even to the level of expert, it is important to maintain a perspective about priorities. C.S. Lewis once wrote "Humility is not thinking less of yourself, it's thinking of yourself less." Be generous with your teaching, share your knowledge and skill without reservation, and do not treat others as lesser based on your own perceived status as a teacher or expert.

Teaching Yoga is teaching. To create a viable and effective teaching environment there must be guidance of behavior on both the student's part and the teacher's part. Standards of behavior create an environment that allows for effective instructor-student communication to occur. Structured communication is required to carry out the often difficult task of teaching someone how to do a challenging physical skill such as a yoga posture.

The fact that a student, a consumer, would choose you to teach them is a privilege which should never be disregarded or forgotten. They have placed a value (paid money) based upon their perception of your knowledge and your ability to provide services. If you create the learning environment appropriately and you do your job correctly, using the tools at hand to improve your student's fitness, health, and happiness, you will have earned the trust, good will, and money given to you. When you teach in a way which does not attend to the basic tenants of professionalism and ethical behavior, you are short-changing your students and denying them the benefits you could have otherwise delivered and for which they compensated you. You are effectively limiting your student's development and denying yourself opportunities for growth, both personally and commercially. The Sanskrit term most closely aligned to this ethic is Ishvarapranidana.

Exercise Professional Ethics

It should be recognized up front that there are virtually no present and binding government regulations on exercise professional behaviors and practices. This means that any exercise profession, including yoga, is self-regulating and self-policing. As such there is a spectrum of codes of ethical behavior available for review and adoption. It is most common to adopt the code of ethics from the major professional association specific to the exercise system in which your practice occurs. For example, the Yoga Alliance, one of the largest international bodies, has adopted a code of ethics that they expect their members and associated instructors to follow (visit their website wwwyogaalliance.org to get a copy).

Adopting the code of the largest and most visible organization has benefits, as in the very unfortunate instance of an ethical complaint against you or your business ending up in some type of litigation. If your actions are within the code of ethics of a large and recognized professional body, the likelihood of a complaint being upheld is smaller. Note that the code of ethics and evidence of your compliance with it must be in evidence. This latter point should not be an issue as good business practice and consumer service is best served through ethical business and personal operations.

There are also smaller and regional organizations with codes of ethical behavior. There can be dozens of competing organizations within the same country. A cautionary note: even though some of the organizations use the same basic name, they may not be affiliated with each other.

While ethics codes may be similar across the discipline, it is best to follow the most robust and consumer friendly system of ethics, as it will satisfy any organization's code of lowers standards.

Codes of ethics may also vary by the nature of the yoga practice. A general public practice may have somewhat different standards that that of a business that is specifically therapeutic in function. An example of this can be seen with the Australian Association of Yoga Therapists Code of Conduct (visit their website at www.yogatherapy.org to obtain a copy of their code of ethics).

It is also prudent to consider the codes of ethics and conduct of other exercise professional bodies. It is generally good practice to be familiar with the codes of the major academic and professional exercise associations and how they relate to your practice. Yoga is exercise and standards of ethical behavior in all exercise professions share a great deal in common. The exercise professional organization most commonly considered to be "authoritative" (based on its 1954 origin and close links to academia and medicine) is the American College of Sports Medicine (visit their website at www.acsm.org to obtain a copy of their code of ethics).

There are hundreds of other exercise associations and organizations—charity, not-for-profit, for profit, educational, spiritual, and sporting—that will have their own twists on ethical codes.

It is important that your adopted code fit the scope of your practice, and most importantly, it must protect the trainee (the consumer) and the trainer (you as the contracted professional). We must also look at the larger picture. As yoga is a system of exercise, it is prudent to consider the standards for professional ethics that are applicable in individual yoga practice, fitness and exercise businesses, and the court. The take home point here is that when it comes to ethical codes, you must have one and you must follow it. The basic tenets of yoga demand no less.

"The main goal in life careerwise should always
be to try to get paid to simply be yourself."

Kevin Smith

SECTION 2 – LEARNING BASIC YOGA POSTURES

"Always doing what you are told doesn't mean you will succeed in life."

Jiro

Deconstructing Yoga is a book for people who want to learn yoga and people who want to teach it. The physical sphere of yoga is the foundation on which every other aspect of yoga practice is built. Addressing the physical basis of yoga first, as we do in this book, will give anyone unparalleled preparation to learn and experience the deeper elements more quickly, efficiently, and completely through later instruction.

Mastering this material on a personal level will help you become a more effective yoga practitioner and prepare you to take full advantage of the teaching you have received in the past and may receive in the present or future. Furthermore, it will make you a more informed customer, enabling you to make educated judgments about the quality of your instructor(s) and instruction material.

For beginners, learning correct technique and procedures in detail at the outset of a fitness journey will pay dividends for years after.

For professionals and aspiring professionals, the meaty, no-filler guides and techniques presented here provide a foundation for developing an effective practice.

It is incumbent upon all fitness professionals to learn and demonstrate the exercises and skills that they will ultimately teach. This goes back to the old saying "if you're gonna talk the talk, ya' better walk the walk." This book has complete and straight-forward instructions to teach you how to teach and how to program. Perhaps most importantly, it also has thorough and effective strategies on how to do.

From the student perspective, a yoga instructor's body is a living version of a PowerPoint™ presentation. Instructors need to consider their own bodies as part of their teaching toolboxes.

For those learning postures for the first time who do not have access to personal instruction, the following section includes extensively illustrated, step-by-step instructions on moving into the postures. For those that want to use or teach yoga as part of a broadly scoping strategy to improve mobility and health, the descriptions within provide an excellent learning and teaching base that is reinforced by the Learning and Teaching Checklist included at the end of each individual posture's presentation.

To make learning and teaching yoga approachable, we present the postures in "triplet form." Three postures are linked together in common purpose to increase mobility in a joint or set of joints. This enables you to easily select a triplet to include for targeted mobility work after a training session and it provides you a simple means of creating a stand-alone range of motion session by selecting multiple triplets. Both of these approaches improve the range-of-motion, balance, and coordination components of mobility and have a direct benefit in application through enabling proper exercise.

The functional organization of each triplet is:

1. Three postures targeting specific joints or regions,
2. Each posture is held for thirty seconds,
3. Each posture is repeated three times.

With all these threes, the triplet system is both functional and easy to remember.

Moving into a Posture

When moving into a posture there is a defined sequence of events.

The first element is a vital one: to establish the foundation of support. Whether it is on the feet, knees, butt, back, arms, or hands, the foundation dictates the stability of the posture and the capacity of the practitioner to assume it.

The second element is to achieve the proper alignment and extension of the body or body parts to produce the required joint extensions and position(s). This element may require several intermediary steps.

The third and final element is to engage in any rotational movements. Again, this element may require several intermediary steps.

It can often be a cue to remember the following word sequence in order to aid the assumption of postures in the correct order of movement:

Foundation – Lengthen – Rotation

A Primer in Breathing

Breathing is important and although there is a complete branch of Yoga, Pranayama, that considers and develops respiratory control and function, we can take baby steps to get started. When we begin learning the physical postures of Yoga, there are just a few things to remember.

Each posture presented requires proper breathing. Traditionally each inhalation is through the nose and each exhalation is through the nose (the restricted airway diameter for nasal inhalation requires higher muscular effort; the larger airway diameter for oral exhalation requires less muscular effort). Each inhalation should take three seconds and each exhalation should take three seconds. Five such breathing cycles result in a thirty second duration, the perfect target time for holding each posture.

Breathing cycles are often linked to flexion and extension; exhalation during flexion, inhalation during extension. When moving in and out of a posture that involves the hips or the shoulders, focused, effective breathing is a priority; the following explains why.

Flexion at the hip, especially as it approaches maximal range of motion, causes compression of the abdominal cavity. This contributes to easy expiration of the breath. Extension of the shoulders, or raising the arms overhead, increases thoracic cavity space, or volume, and aids in complete inhalation.

In general, as the hips straighten through extension or as the arms are extended overhead, inhale; as the hips flex forward or the arms are lowered, exhale. In this way breathing is linked to movement.

"We keep moving forward, opening new doors, and doing new things, because we're curious and curiosity keeps leading us down new paths."

Walt Disney

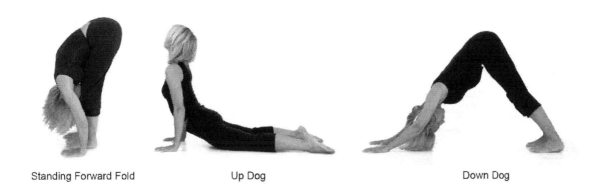

Standing Forward Fold   Up Dog   Down Dog

Standing Forward Fold   ~ Uttanasana ~

Fitness gurus often ask if you can touch your toes. Can you? The Standing Forward Fold is a warm up posture and flexibility developer for the hamstrings and vertebral column. Sometimes this posture is confused with simply telling someone to touch their toes. The Forward Fold, unlike the simpler "touch the toes" position, limits upper and lower vertebral rounding and therefore more fully develops the range of motion of the hamstrings.

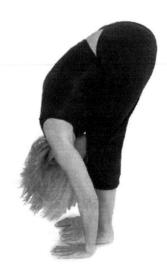

How to do it

1. Standing at the front of the mat with feet hip width apart, knees over toes, spread the feet over the mat making sure the four smaller toes of each foot are together and the big toe is spread as far out as possible while remaining comfortable.

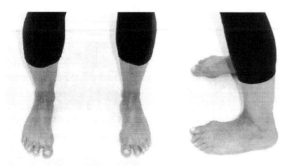

NOTE: As proficiency builds, the stance is narrowed until the medial borders of the feet are touching.

2. Lift your hands above your head, palms together. Tilt back the head and look at your hands.
3. Fold (or bend) forward from the hip joints, bringing your arms down towards the floor. Make sure your knees are soft (slightly bent) as you go down. If your hamstrings are tight, bend your knees more.

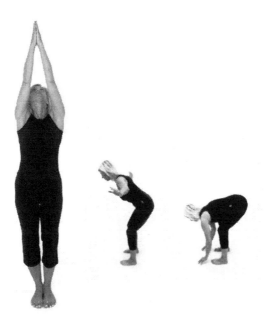

4. Allow your head to lower down toward the floor. Relax the vertebral column. Now lift your shoulders away from the floor, making sure the scapula is in neutral position. A guide for head position is to look at the end of your mat.
5. Let the head hang towards the floor.

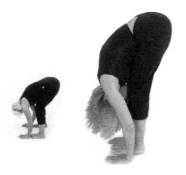

> **NOTE:** Once the initial fold is completed, in either the beginner's shoulder width or desired narrow stance, the hands move to the sides of the feet and the knees are gently extended.

6. Each time you exhale, make sure you bring your body a little closer into your thighs. With each exhale, feel the rib cage rest securely and comfortably against the thighs. With each exhalation, also bring the chin in towards the neck. This will fully extend the cervical region of the neck.

7. Gently shift your balance forward and feel your weight coming toward your toes. As you do this, attempt to pull the navel up and into (back towards) the vertebral column and, if you can, rest your hands flat on the floor directly beside your feet.

8. Hold for five breath cycles.

9. Recover back to the starting position. Come up slowly on a single deep, slow, and controlled inhalation. Keep your knees slightly bent and roll through your vertebral column slowly, from bottom to top (lumbar – thoracic – cervical), in order to return to the standing start position. When you exit postures in the future, use this method to return to standing position.

10. Finish with the arms resting at your sides.

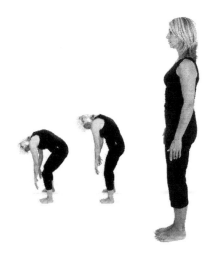

What are the benefits?

1. Develops range of motion around the hip by stretching the hamstrings (semitendinosus, semimembranosus, and biceps femoris) and gluteals.

2. Develops range of motion (flexion) along the individual joints of the vertebral column.

3. Is soothing to the nervous system (relaxing).
4. When included as a part of a training sequence, this posture aids in the reduction of anxiety, depression, and perceived stress.
5. With straighter knee position, the calves (gastrocnemius, soleus) will also be stretched.
6. In beginning trainees, strengthens the muscles supporting the arches of the feet, the knees and the thighs.
7. Has been reported to relieve discomfort associated with menopause.
8. Can increase gastric motility.
9. Develops local muscular endurance in all muscles actively contracting in the posture.

Contraindications

This is a very low risk exercise position. However, individuals with orthopaedic problems of the back may be at risk of injury and should consult a physician before participating. It is possible to reduce back stress during the exercise by not bending forwards fully and by keeping the knees slightly bent. Modification can be made for pregnancy by using a wider foot stance and keeping knees bent. As with any exercise movement requiring balance, caution must be exercised with individuals with active ear infections, other eye/ear conditions affecting balance or orthostatic intolerance (moving the head from an inferior position to a superior position—standing up-causing dizziness).

Learning and Teaching Check List

1. Is the foundation, or body mass, distributed across the feet equally?   ◯
2. Do the ribs progressively get closer and closer to the thighs?   ◯
3. Is the trainee's body mass slowly moving forward toward the toes?   ◯
4. Are the trainee's knees extended to near the limit of extension?   ◯
5. Are the trainee's shoulders extended and relaxed?   ◯
6. Is the trainee's neck relaxed?   ◯
7. Are the ischial tuberosities pointing at the ceiling and not the wall?   ◯
8. Are the elbows relaxed and not forcefully locked out and struggling to reach?   ◯
9. Is the trainee breathing throughout?   ◯
10. Does the trainee hold the final position for five full breath cycles?   ◯

Up Dog   ~ Urdhva Mukha Svanasana ~

This is a stretch of the entire anterior face of the body. It is often perceived as a "back bend." Up Dog is the opposing, complementary posture to Down Dog (next), which stretches the entire posterior musculature of the body. For this reason both poses are generally included in early sections of yoga training sessions.

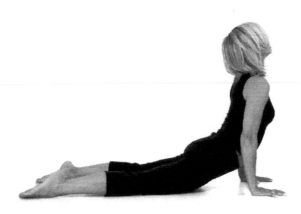

How to do it

1. From the Plank posture (top of a Push-Up position), slowly flex (bend) the elbows until they are a little lower than 90°. This is referred to as "lower plank posture."
2. Lower the legs until the anterior (front) of the thighs are just off of the floor.

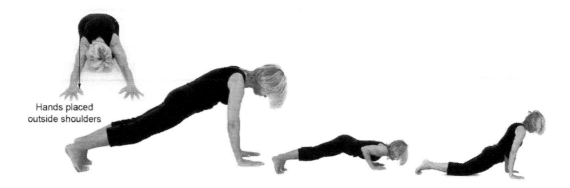

Hands placed
outside shoulders

3. The feet should roll forward from their support position on the balls of the feet to a point where the entire top of the foot is in contact with the floor.

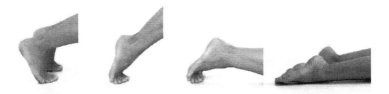

4. The quadriceps (rectus femoris, vastus medialis, vastus lateralis, vastus intermedus) should be engaged to generate force between the top of the feet and the floor. This will lift the upper thighs off the floor.
5. Take a deep breath and retract the scapulae (tense the rhomboideus muscles to pull the shoulder blades to midline).
6. Extend the elbows (push up) while lifting the chest up (arch the back) and slightly lifting the chin to extend the cervical vertebrae.
7. Slowly look up and roll the head back until the occipital portion of the skull (back) is near the top of the trapezius (top of shoulders) and creates a stretch on the anterior of the neck.
8. Tense the rectus abdominis and pull it towards the vertebral column.
9. Relax as much of the posterior musculature as possible.
10. Hold for five breath cycles.

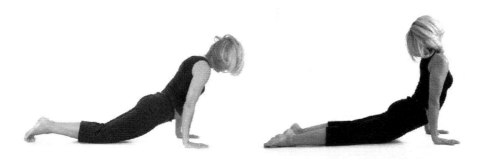

What are the benefits?

1. Improves mobility (degree of extension) around the hip and the vertebral column.
2. Improves posture and carriage of the vertebral column, chest, and shoulders.

3. When included as a part of a training sequence, this posture aids in the reduction of anxiety, depression, and perceived stress.
4. Develops local muscular endurance in all muscles actively contracting in the posture.

Contraindications

The primary issue preventing participation in this posture is any wrist or hand pathology such as carpal tunnel syndrome or advanced arthritis. Pregnancy, especially in the 2nd and 3rd trimesters will preclude use of this posture.

Learning and Teaching Check List

1. Are the trainee's toes and tops of the feet flat on the floor? ◯
2. Are the trainee's upper thighs suspended off the floor? ◯
3. Is the pelvis suspended off (not touching) the floor and the iliac crest tilted toward the floor? ◯
4. Are the hands placed just outside or barely under the shoulders? ◯
5. Are the elbows extended near anatomical limit but not completely locked out? ◯
6. Are the shoulders (scapulae and acromioclavicular joints) pulled down and back? ◯
7. Is the head tilted upwards thus giving the entire body a sweeping backward arch? ◯
8. Is the trainee breathing throughout? ◯
9. Does the trainee hold the final position for five full breath cycles? ◯

Down Dog   ~ Adho Mukha Svanasana ~

This is a stretch of the entire posterior of the body. This posture resembles an inverted "v" when done properly. Down Dog stretches the entire posterior musculature of the body and is complementary to Up Dog (previous). For this reason both poses are generally included in early sections of yoga training sessions.

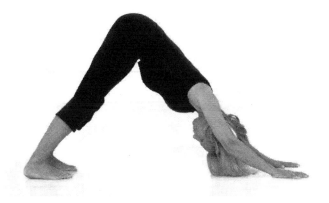

How to do it

1. Start on the floor on hands and knees in the Table position. Your toes should be pointed directly backwards.

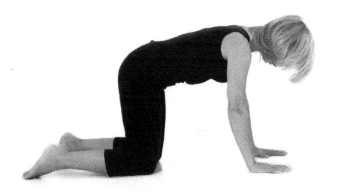

NOTE: The Table posture is described in the Beginnings & Endings Chapter.

2. Flex at the knees and move the ischial tuberosities (butt bones) back until they are resting upon the heels (calcaneous bones of both feet). This will place your feet at roughly hip width, the desired width between the feet of the final posture.

3. Stretch the arms straight forward, palms down, as far as you can reach. The hands should be directly in front of the shoulder joints (not too narrow or too wide). The fingers should be spread to improve the area of floor contact to ensure stability of position.

4. The forehead should be facing the floor.

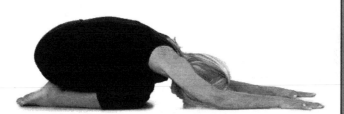

> **NOTE:** This intermediate posture is called the Child's Pose (Balasana) and should be remembered as it will be useful on future occasions. In this particular use, it will define the correct distance that the hands should be away from the feet in this posture – based on individual height and limb lengths.

5. Without moving the hands or knees, lift your feet and bring the toes under the heels.

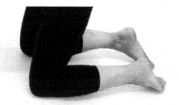 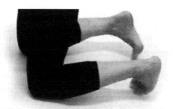 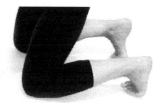

6. Raise the hips into the air by extending the knees (straighten the legs). As the hips rise, push the feet into the floor so the heels are down but slightly off the floor. The balls of the feet should touch the floor and carry the body weight. The toes do not carry weight here and you should be able to lift them off the floor as a test of this.

7. Straighten the leg so that the ankle, knee, and hip form a straight line that is roughly at a right angle ($90°$) to a line formed by the hand, elbow, shoulder and hip–the inverted "v"–with the ischial tuberosities forming the point of the "v". The wrist joint will be extended (bent back) at about $30°$. The elbow and shoulder joints should be pushing toward their complete range of motion. This requires muscular exertion and forms the stimulus for improvements in range of motion and local muscular fitness. If you can fully extend a joint to its anatomical limit already, leave the joint slightly

unlocked to ensure that the appropriate musculature is recruited; fully locked joints require very little muscular effort to maintain position.

8. Lifting the chest will place the lumbar and thoracic vertebrae in normal extension. The cervical spine (neck) should also be held in normal extension. This means that the ears should be roughly between the elbows and the line of sight should somewhere at knee level or above.

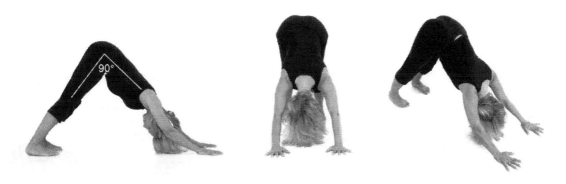

NOTE: Certain viewpoints are better than others for detecting and correcting technique. A good instructor will look at the trainee from multiple positions

9. Initially, it may be difficult to achieve one of the straight lines or both. If it is difficult to extend the knee with the heel near the floor, it is acceptable to keep the knee bent and progressively attempt to straighten it over time. Alternatively the heel can be raised to enable full knee extension and then the gastrocnemius and soleus muscles (calf muscles) can be relaxed over time to allow full range of motion and almost full foot contact. If the back rounds or the shoulders initially do not come into alignment, the chest should be pushed down towards the floor and the scapulae (shoulder blades) should be retracted and depressed (pulled towards midline and down) to establish a straighter position.

10. In the final position, the abdominal musculature contracts and pulls in towards the vertebral column.

11. Hold for five breath cycles.

What are the benefits?

1. Develops range of motion (flexion) around the hip by stretching the hamstrings (semitendinosus, semimembranosus, and biceps femoris) and gluteals.
2. Develops range of motion (dorsiflexion) around the ankle by stretching the gastrocnemious, soleus, and plantaris.
3. Develops the shoulder in extension by isometrically loading the long head of the biceps brachii, latissimus dorsi, pectoralis major, and posterior deltoid.
4. Develops the back musculature in extension by isometrically loading the erectors spinae, trapezius, rhomboideus, and latissimus dorsi.
5. When included as a part of a training sequence, this posture aids in the reduction of anxiety, depression, and perceived stress.
6. In beginning trainees, strengthens the muscles supporting the arches of the feet, the knees, hips, vertebrae, shoulders, elbows, wrists, and hands.
7. Improves midline musculoskeletal stability.
8. Develops local muscular endurance in all muscles actively contracting in the posture.

Contraindications

Due to the body weight being supported on them, any orthopedic issues with the hands and wrists (such as carpal tunnel syndrome) may preclude performing this posture. Due to the inverted nature of this posture, those with chronic headaches, diagnosed hypertension, active inner ear infections, or orthostatic intolerance should approach this posture with caution.

Learning and Teaching Check List

1. Is the trainee's foundation, or body mass, distributed across the hands and feet equally? ○
2. Is their body weight on the balls of their feet and their heels near the floor? ○
3. Are the patellas pointing down and forward? ○
4. Are the ischial tuberosities pointed up with the body in an upside down "v," not a "u"? ○
5. Is the neck in normal extension and the head not aimed excessively up or down? ○
6. Is the trainee breathing throughout? ○
7. Does the trainee hold the final position for five full breath cycles? ○

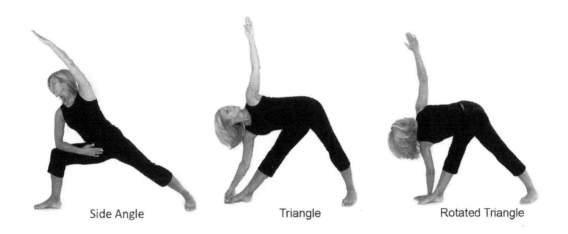

Side Angle   Triangle   Rotated Triangle

Side Angle   ~ Utthita Parsvakonasana ~

This is a potent wide-stance side, adductor, and hamstring stretch that is suitable for virtually all populations.

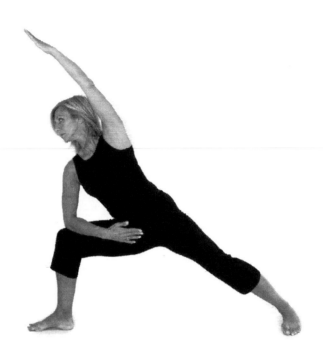

How to do it

1. Begin by standing in Mountain posture (see Beginning & Endings for description).
2. Step back with one foot (in these illustrations, the left is used). This foot is now the trailing foot. Keep the knee of the other leg (the lead) bent at slightly greater than 90°. This is now the leading leg. Keep the leading knee in line with the leading ankle.
3. Rotate the trailing foot outwards approximately 45°. Stand with the torso facing perpendicular to the lead foot.
4. For beginners the distance between front and back feet should be far enough apart to feel a mild stretch in the thighs. For experienced trainees the feet should be

spaced about 1½ leg lengths apart (this could be more than 4 feet in long legged individuals).

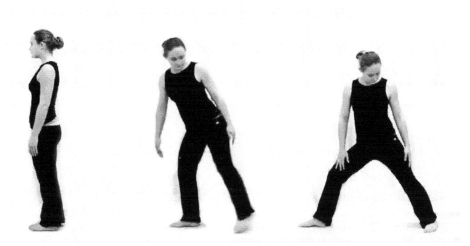

5. The torso should be facing to the open side (not towards the toes of the lead foot). Lean the torso over the lead leg. This is a version of the side bend. Bring the lateral aspect of the rib cage towards the top of the leading leg's thigh.

6. Complete the torso lean by placing the arm on the same side of the lead leg on top of the knee, within a few inches of the top of the patella. The elbow should touch the leg but the arm should not be used as a support for the upper bodyweight; the abdominal and thoracic musculature should be used to hold position.

7. Abduct the trailing arm up over the head until it is on the same line as the torso.

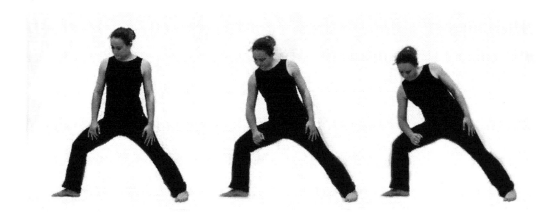

8. The arm should be internally rotated so the hand can be placed, palm inwards, on the medial and proximal thigh of the lead leg. The fingers should be in contact with the anterior surface of the lower abdomen.
9. Pull the hips under the torso. When viewed from above, the body from foot to hand should roughly be in a straight line.
10. Ensure that the lumbar, thoracic and cervical vertebrae are in normal extension. For an additional torsional element, turn the head to look up at the trailing inner elbow or ceiling.
11. Hold for five breath cycles.
12. Reverse the process to exit the posture and repeat on the opposing side.

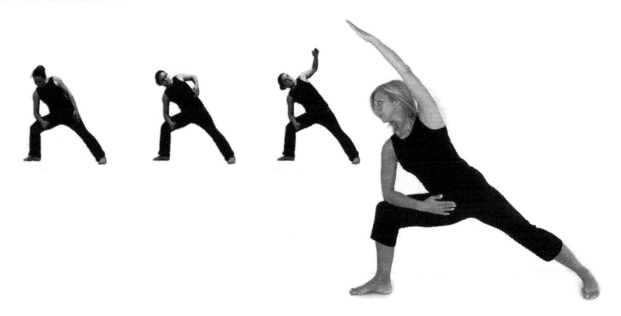

What are the benefits?

1. Improves balance, coordination, and posture.
2. Improves range of motion through stretching of the hips (adductors - adductor brevis, adductor longus, adductor magnus, pectineus, and gracilis; extensors - semitendinosus, semimembranosus, and biceps femoris), back (latissimus dorsi, quadratus lumborum), lateral abdomen (externus obliquus, internus obliquus), and lateral thorax (intercostalis, serratus anterior).

3. For beginners, provides a strength stimulus for the quadriceps (rectus femoris, vastus medialis, vastus lateralis, vastus intermedus) and gluteals.
4. When included as a part of a training sequence, this posture aids in the reduction of anxiety, depression, and perceived stress.
5. Develops local muscular endurance in all muscles actively contracting in the posture.

Contraindications

While this is a somewhat difficult posture to attain correctly, it is a low risk movement. There is no orthostatic challenge and only a minor increase in non-contraction induced resistance to blood flow (one arm overhead). Individuals with diagnosed hip, knee, or neck pathologies may require modification or may wish to not participate in the posture.

Learning and Teaching Checklist

1. Are the trainee's feet spread widely apart forward to back?   ○
2. Is the lead foot straight ahead and the lead leg also forward and bent slightly above 90° at the knee?   ○
3. Is the trailing leg straight with the foot flat on the floor and pointed laterally?   ○
4. Torso moved into final position via lateral tilt?   ○
5. Is the elbow on the lead knee with hand on upper thigh and abdomen?   ○
6. Do the trailing leg, torso, and overhead arm form an approximate 45° straight line, hand to floor?   ○
7. Is the trainee breathing throughout?   ○
8. Does the trainee hold the final position for five full breath cycles?   ○

Triangle   ~ Utthita Trikonasana ~

The Triangle posture is a wide-stance side bend that develops range of motion around the hip and low back. It is a simpler, anterior-facing version of the rotated triangle.

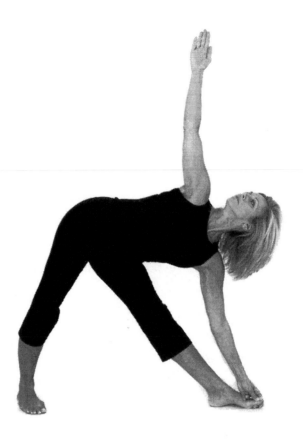

How to do it

1. Begin in Mountain posture (see Beginnings & Endings for description).
2. Rotate the trailing foot outwards approximately 45°. Stand with the torso facing perpendicular to the lead foot.
3. Keep the entire rear foot in contact with the floor.
4. Keep the rear foot flat on the floor and the rear knee extended. Straighten the front knee so both legs are straight and the body is now facing the long side of the mat. The front hip should now be externally rotated and the front foot pointed lateral to the direction of the torso.

5. Raise the arms (abduct them) to where they are parallel to the floor. Fingers should be completely extended and together.

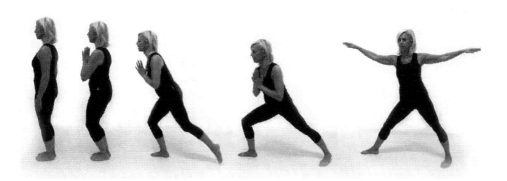

6. Stretch and bend from the front hip; slightly bend the front knee and reach down with the leading hand. Wrap two fingers around the leading big toe (hallux) or four fingers under the lateral border of the foot (or hold the ankle if required). Keep the back in normal extension (don't round it) during this step. The trailing arm and hand should be perpendicular to the floor.
7. Turn the head and look up at the trailing-side hand. Gently retract and depress the scapulae (shoulders back and down).
8. Push gently up by extending (straightening) the lead knee. Beginners and those with poor flexibility will not be able to completely straighten the knee but should push to their limit of flexibility. Blocks can be used to bring the floor to the knee. Note that the knees should be extended by gentle quadriceps contraction in order to produce a controlled hamstring stretch.
9. Engage the abdominal musculature. You should feel like you are attempting to pull your navel back towards the vertebral column.
10. Ideally, in the final position, both arms and the shoulders should be in a nearly straight vertical line.
11. Hold for five breath cycles.
12. Return to the standing posture. Bend the knee slightly to come up, and repeat the above using the opposite side.

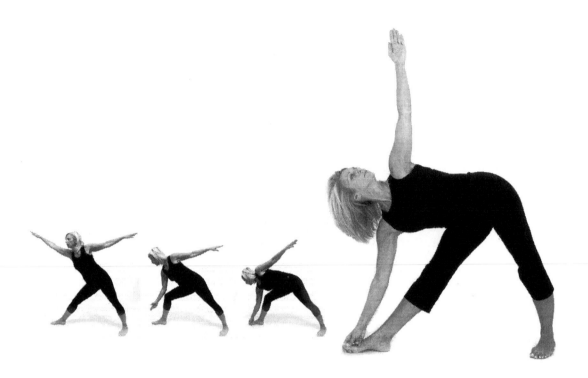

What are the benefits?

1. Improves mobility around the hip of the leading leg by stretching the hamstrings (semitendinosus, semimembranosus, biceps femoris) and gluteals.
2. In beginners, improves rotational strength along the musculature of the lumbar vertebrae (erectors spinae, quatratus lumborum) and abdomen (externus obliquus, internus obliquus).
3. When included as a part of a training sequence, this posture aids in the reduction of anxiety, depression, and perceived stress.
4. Develops local muscular endurance in all muscles actively contracting in the posture.

Contraindications

Those with cervical or lumbar vertebral issues may wish to consider avoiding or modifying this posture. Due to the changes in head height in the assumption of and exit from the posture, those with orthostatic intolerance should exercise caution and move slowly.

Learning and Teaching Checklist

1. Is the lead foot flat and pointed directly outward, trailing foot flat and angled at 45°? ◯
2. Is the same side hand grasping the leading foot's big toe? ◯
3. Is the leading knee as straight as possible and the trailing leg completely straight? ◯
4. Is the trailing arm extended perpendicular to the floor? ◯
5. Are the head and gaze directed up at the trailing (raised) hand? ◯
6. Is the back rotated but held in normal lordotic and kyphotic extension? ◯
7. Is the trainee breathing throughout? ◯
8. Does the trainee hold the final position for five full breath cycles? ◯

Rotated Triangle   ~Parivrtta Trikonasana~

The Rotated Triangle posture is a wide-stance rotated side bend that develops range of motion around the hip and lower back. It is a more challenging, rotated variant of the Triangle posture.

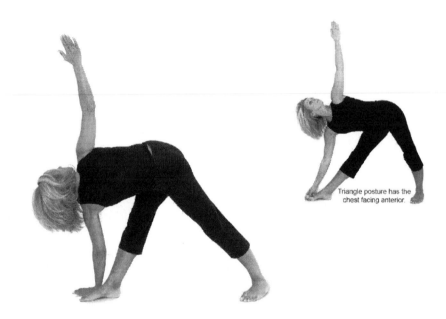

Triangle posture has the chest facing anterior.

Note the difference in torso orientation between the Rotated Triangle (L) and the Triangle (R).

How to do it

1. Begin in Mountain posture.
2. Step one foot back and rotate the trailing foot outwards approximately 45°. Stand with the torso facing perpendicular to the lead foot.
3. Keep the entire rear foot in contact with the floor.

4. Stand with the hips facing perpendicular to the lead foot. Both knees are in extension.
5. Place the hands on the waist just above the hips.
6. Bend forward. Keep the back in normal extension (don't round it) during this step. Reach down with both hands and place the fingertips on the floor slightly in front of the feet.
7. Now lift the torso (via hip extension) until the line of the vertebral column is parallel to the floor. The cervical vertebrae should be in normal extension with the head well away from the shoulders.
8. The body mass should be distributed across both feet.

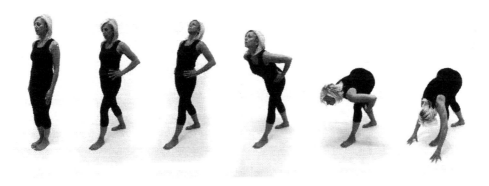

9. Place the trailing-side hand on the floor outside the lead foot. If needed, bend the knees slightly in order to reach the floor, or use a block to bring the floor level up.
10. Place the lead hand on the top of the lead leg. Gently push the hip backward as you rotate the rib cage around toward the leading-side of the mat.
11. When torso rotation is to the limit of range of motion, abduct and extend the lead arm up towards the ceiling. Ideally, in the final position, both arms and the shoulders between should be in a straight vertical line.
12. Turn the head and look up at the elevated hand.
13. During the time in the final posture, push gently up by extending (straightening) the lead knee. Beginners and those with poor flexibility will not be able to completely straighten the knee but should push to their limit of flexibility.

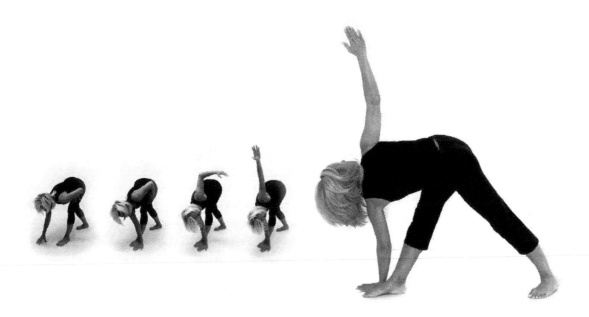

14. Hold for five breath cycles.
15. Return to the standing posture. Bend the knee slightly to come up, and repeat the above using the opposite side.

What are the benefits?

1. Improves mobility around the hip of the leading leg by stretching the hamstrings (semitendinosus, semimembranosus, biceps femoris) and gluteals.
2. In beginners, improves rotational strength along the musculature of the lumbar vertebrae (erectors spinae, quatratus lumborum) and abdomen (externus obliquus, internus obliquus).
3. When included as a part of a training sequence, this posture aids in the reduction of anxiety, depression, and perceived stress.
4. Develops local muscular endurance in all muscles actively contracting in the posture.

Contraindications

Those with cervical or lumbar vertebral issues may wish to consider avoiding or modifying this posture. Due to the changes in head height in the assumption of and exit from the posture, those with orthostatic intolerance should exercise caution and move slowly.

Learning and Teaching Checklist

1. Is the lead foot flat and pointed directly outward, trailing foot flat and angled at 45°? ◯
2. Is the opposite side hand on the floor inside or outside the foot? ◯
3. Is the leading knee as straight as possible, trailing leg completely straight? ◯
4. Is the leading side arm extended upward perpendicular to the floor? ◯
5. Is the trainee's head looking up at the leading hand? ◯
6. Is the back rotated but held in normal kyphotic and lordotic extension? ◯
7. Is the trainee breathing throughout? ◯
8. Does the trainee hold the final position for five full breath cycles? ◯

"Many people find the universe confusing – it's not."

Stephen Hawking

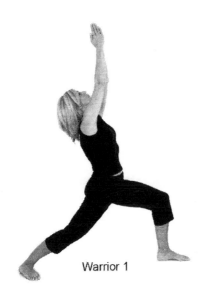

Warrior 1

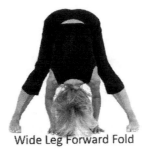

Wide Leg Forward Fold

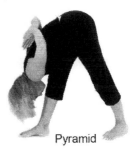

Pyramid

Warrior 1

~ Virabhadrasana 1 ~

This is a standing asymmetric posture that loads the quadriceps of the leading leg and develops mobility of the trailing hip and ankle.

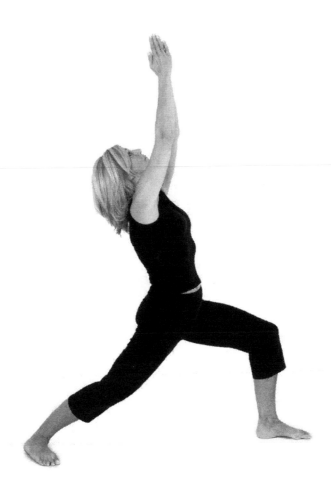

How to do it

1. Begin in Mountain posture.
2. Step backwards with one leg. This is now the trailing leg. This should be a step of two to three feet, less if the step back causes the hips to rotate. Keep the lead foot pointing forward. Rotate the trailing foot approximately 45° (rotate the entire leg to achieve this).

3. Flex (bend) the leading leg until there is an approximate 90° angle between the femur and tibia. The leading knee should be directly over the leading ankle and the foot should be flat on the floor.
4. Fully extend the trailing knee to stretch the anterior hip and push the heel of the trailing foot down to the floor if possible. This will stretch the posterior musculature of the ankle.

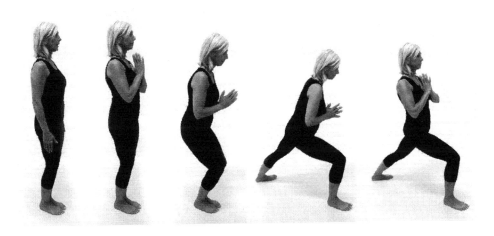

5. Keep the torso and hips facing forward.
6. The vertebral column should be held in normal extension along its length (no excessive arching or rounding).
7. Raise the arms and extend them overhead, biceps pointing toward the ears, palms facing each other and touching if possible.
8. Gently roll the head back (cervical extension) and direct the gaze at the thumbs.
9. Hold for five breath cycles.
10. Return to the standing posture. Bend the knee slightly to come up, and repeat the above using the opposite side.

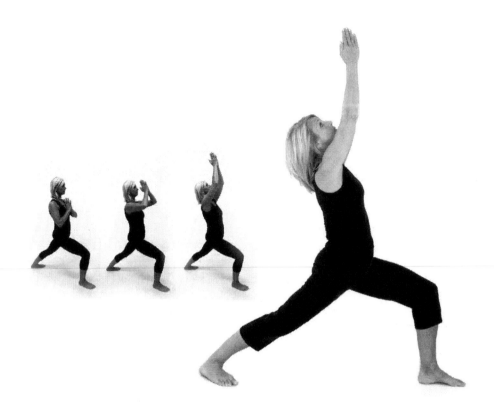

What are the benefits?

1. In beginners, strength can be developed in the quadriceps (rectus femoris, vastus medialis, vastus laterals, vastus internus) and gluteals.
2. Develops range of motion around the hip by stretching the anterior hip musculature (rectus femoris, sartorius).
3. Develops range of motion around the ankle by stretching the related posterior musculature (gastrocnemius, soleus, plantaris).
4. When included as a part of a training sequence, this posture aids in the reduction of anxiety, depression, and perceived stress.
5. Develops local muscular endurance in all muscles actively contracting in the posture.

Contraindications

This is a low risk posture. Individuals with existing hip injury or disease may wish to not participate or modify the position. There is increased vascular resistance to blood flow via raised arms that might be of concern to someone with diagnosed heart disease.

Learning and Teaching Checklist

1. Is the lead foot flat on the floor? ○
2. Is the lead ankle directly below the knee and the knee angle approximating 90°? ○
3. Are both hips facing forward (minimal twisting)? ○
4. Is the trailing knee extended? ○
5. Is the trailing foot's heel on the floor or actively being pushed down? ○
6. Is the back held in normal kyophotic and lordotic vertebral extension? ○
7. Are the arms overhead, elbows extended, and palms together? ○
8. Is the chest up and shoulders back and down? ○
9. Is the head tilted up and the gaze directed upward? ○
10. Is the trainee breathing throughout? ○
11. Does the trainee hold the final position for five full breath cycles? ○

Wide Leg Forward Fold   ~ Prasarita Padottanasana ~

This is a standing, wide-based posture that strongly develops range of motion around the posterior of the hips.

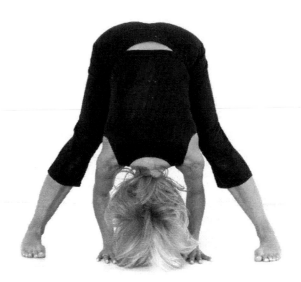

How to do it

1. Begin in Mountain posture.
2. Step with one foot laterally. This should be a wide step out, approximately three to four feet depending on leg length (short legs – closer to three feet; long legs – closer to four feet).
3. Keep the toes pointed directly forward and the feet parallel to each other. The bodyweight should be evenly distributed across the soles of the feet. The toes should be lifted off the floor slightly. This will place equal pressure on the balls of the feet and the heels. Gently contract the quadriceps to extend the knee and engage a posterior stretch on the hamstrings.
4. The knees should be held in gentle extension throughout the posture.
5. Place the hands on the hips at a level above the iliac crest (top of hip bone).

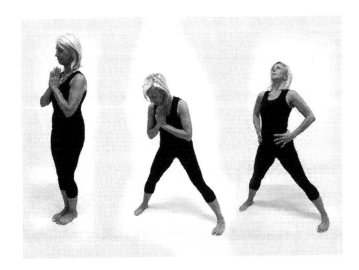

6. While maintaining the vertebral column in normal extension, bend forward (flex) at the hips and begin slowly lowering the head and shoulders toward the floor.

7. Touch the floor with your fingertips as you near the end of your range of motion (do not round the shoulders and back to make this happen). Continue on and place your palms on the floor. If you cannot touch the floor with extended knees and the back in normal extension, flex the knees enough to get your fingers on the floor. Then push up with the knees to try to extend the knees as far as you can (this will likely be the position in which beginners and those with poor flexibility will initially end).

8. Continue to lower the torso forward (you can let gravity help by relaxing the posterior hip musculature) until the torso is suspended upside-down and nearly vertical below the hips and in between the legs. You can use the heel of your hands to push against the floor and push the torso backwards towards the heels. If possible, the head should be touching the floor just forward of a line between the toes of the right and left feet.

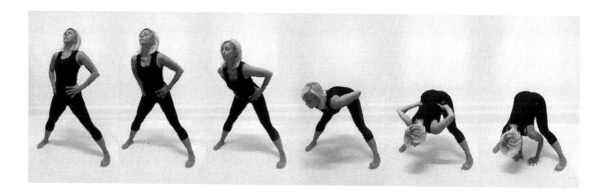

9. The hands should end flat on the floor under the shoulders and along a line between the right and left heels. The fingers should be pointing forward. The forearms will be nearly vertical and the upper arm nearly parallel to the floor. The elbows should be pointing back and under the hips, not to the side. This helps keep the shoulders in a neutral position.

10. The scapulae should be gently squeezed to the midline. The neck should be relaxed with no significant weight placed on the head. The head should be easy to move from side to side.

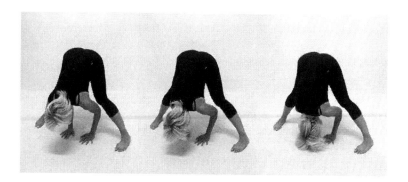

11. Hold for five breath cycles.

What are the benefits?

1. Provides a significant stretching stimulus to the hamstrings (semitendinosus, semimembranosus, and biceps femoris), the adductors (adductor brevis, adductor longus, adductor magnus, pectineus, and gracilis), and the gastrocnemius.

2. When included as a part of a training sequence, this posture aids in the reduction of anxiety, depression, and perceived stress.
3. Develops local muscular endurance in all muscles actively contracting in the posture.

Contraindications

Individuals with diagnosed hip or low back problems may wish to avoid this posture. As the head makes significant excursions above and below the heart while moving in and out of this posture, those who are intolerant of orthostatic challenge may also wish to avoid this posture.

Learning and Teaching Checklist

1. Are the feet spread apart and pointed forward?   ◯
2. Are the knees extended?   ◯
3. Is the stretch induced by flexion at the hip, not vertebral rounding?   ◯
4. Does the torso hang easily and vertically in between the legs?   ◯
5. Does the head hang near the floor or touching the floor?   ◯
6. Are the palms on the floor just below and outside the shoulders?   ◯
7. Is the trainee breathing throughout?   ◯
8. Does the trainee hold the final position for five full breath cycles?   ◯

Pyramid

~ Parsvottanasana ~

This is a very potent wide stance side, adductor, and hamstring stretch.

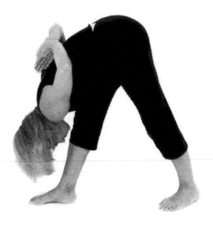

How to do it

1. Begin in Mountain posture.
2. Extend the arms to the rear, behind the back (hands at the level of the hips). Internally rotate the arms at the shoulders and place the hands back-to-back, palms out. This will rotate the shoulder joints slightly forward and the palms will be facing outwards (laterally with thumbs pointing to the rear away from the body).
3. Engage the abdominal musculature. You should feel like you are attempting to pull your navel back towards the vertebral column.
4. Move the hands towards the midline behind the back. Bend the elbows and extend the wrists upwards so the fingers, then the palms, come together behind the back. The lateral border of the hand and fingers will be, or should be, in contact with the lower thoracic vertebrae. The palms should be together. If this is a difficult position to assume, it is appropriate to use an alternative hold where the forearms cross the body and the elbows are grasped by the opposite hand.

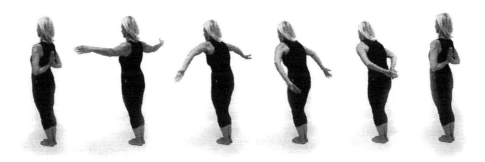

> **NOTE**: For those with limited range of motion or those with larger than average back muscle mass, the hands can be clasped behind the back with the elbows extended.

5. Take a step to the rear with one foot. The step should be relative to leg length, but no more than two feet. The trailing foot should be at an approximate 45° angle (rotate the leg to achieve this).
6. Extend the torso at the hip (lean back slightly).
7. Flex (bend) the trailing knee slightly to lower the body towards the leading foot. Keep lowering the body until the ribs are near or in contact with the leading thigh.
8. Extend the trailing knee gently to push the top of the leading hip up so both hips are parallel with the ceiling.
9. Keep the torso extended (lumbar and thoracic vertebrae in normal extension) over the front leg.

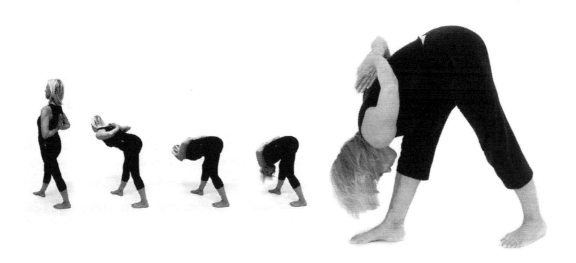

10. Hold for five breath cycles.
11. Without changing arm position behind the body, return to Mountain posture then repeat the sequence on the opposite side.

What are the benefits?

1. Improves balance, coordination, and posture.
2. Improves range of motion through stretching of the hips (extensors - semitendinosus, semimembranosus, and biceps femoris), back (latissimus dorsi, quadratus lumborum), rotator cuff (supraspinatus, infraspinatus, teres minor, subscapularis).
3. For beginners, provides a strength stimulus for the quadriceps (rectus femoris, vastus medialis, vastus lateralis, vastus intermedus), gluteals, and erectors spinae.
4. When included as a part of a training sequence, this posture aids in the reduction of anxiety, depression, and perceived stress.
5. Develops local muscular endurance in all muscles actively contracting in the posture.

Contraindications

While this is a somewhat difficult posture to attain correctly; it is a low risk movement. There is an orthostatic challenge such that those with orthostatic intolerance should use caution with participation. Individuals with diagnosed hip or shoulder pathologies may require modification or may wish to not participate in the posture.

Learning and Teaching Checklist

1. Are the trainee's feet spread approximately two feet apart? ○
2. Is the leading leg extended to near end range of motion? ○ ○
3. Is the trailing leg straight with the foot rotated out about 45° and flat on the floor? ○
4. Are the arms behind the back, internally rotated, with correct hand position? ○
5. Does the torso tilt below parallel to the floor, forward and laterally, with normal vertebral extension? ○
6. Is the trainee breathing throughout? ○
7. Does the trainee hold the final position for five full breath cycles? ○

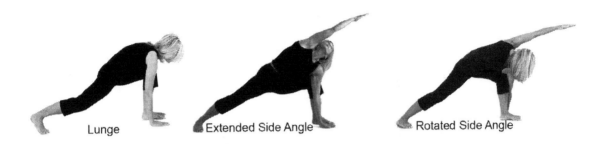

Lunge   Extended Side Angle   Rotated Side Angle

Lunge   ~ No Sanskrit Term ~

The lunge is a kneeling posture that rigorously stretches the anterior and posterior hip musculature.

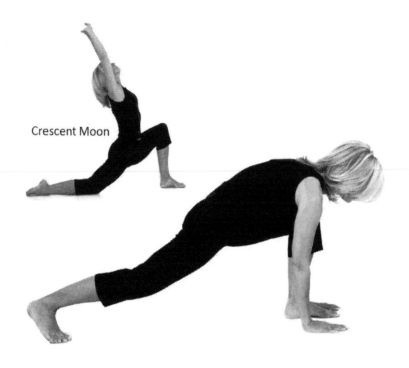

Crescent Moon

How to do it

1. Begin in Mountain posture.
2. Raise the hands above the head, elbows extended as much as possible, biceps facing the ears, and palms together if possible.
3. Bend forward into Forward Fold (refer to description in Triplet 1).
4. Look up, extend the spine, hands flat on the floor.
5. Step back with one foot. Keep the lead knee at 90° and the knee in line with the ankle.
6. Rest hands flat on either side of the front leg.
7. Tuck the chin in and keep the gaze directed at the floor.

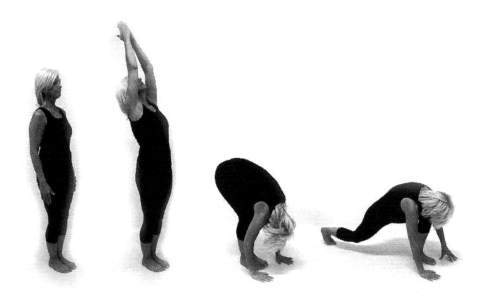

8. Hold for five breath cycles.
9. Return to standing position then repeat the sequence with the opposite side.
10. As range of motion improves the Lunge can be modified to an arms-overhead position called the Crescent Moon (see inset in first image).

What are the benefits?

1. Improved range of motion in the hips via stretching of the hamstrings (semitendinosus, semimembranosus, and biceps femoris), adductors (adductor brevis, adductor longus, adductor magnus, pectineus, and gracilis), gluteals, and sartorius.
2. In beginners, strength can be developed in the gluteals, erector spinae, and quadriceps (rectus femoris, vastus lateralis, vastus medialis, vastus internus).
3. When included as a part of a training sequence, this posture aids in the reduction of anxiety, depression, and perceived stress.
4. Develops local muscular endurance in all muscles actively contracting in the posture.

Contraindications

As this posture begins with the head below the hips and with the head above the hips in the final posture, individuals sensitive to orthostatic challenge may need to refrain from participation. Individuals with diagnosed hip or knee problems may need to forgo participation or use a modification.

Learning and Teaching Checklist

1. Is the leading foot flat on the floor and pointed straight forward?
2. Is the leading knee over the lead foot?
3. Are the trailing shin, top of foot, and toes on the floor directly to the rear?
4. Are the hips lower than the leading knee?
5. Is the low back gently arched thus allowing the upper body to be vertical?
6. Is the head tilted towards the floor?
7. Is the trainee breathing throughout?
8. Does the trainee hold the final position for five full breath cycles?

○
○
○
○
○
○
○
○

Extended Side Angle   ~ Utthita Parsvakonasana ~

This is a very potent standing wide-stance side, adductor, and hamstring stretch. It is the slightly simpler cousin of the Rotated Side Angle.

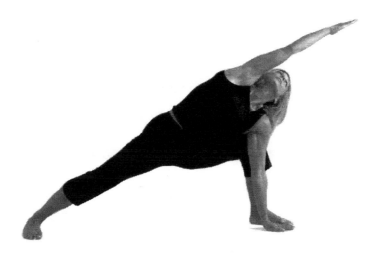

How to do it

1. Begin in Mountain posture.
2. Raise the hands above the head, elbows extended as much as possible, biceps facing the ears, and palms together if possible.
3. Bend forward into Forward Fold (refer to description in Triplet 1).
4. Look up and extend the spine, hands flat on the floor.
5. Step back with one foot; keep the lead knee at 90° and knee in line with the ankle. Rest hands flat on either side of the lead leg to keep balance during foot placement.
6. For beginners the feet should be far enough apart to feel a mild stretch in the thighs. For experienced trainees the feet should be spaced about 1½ leg lengths apart (this could be more than 4 feet in long legged individuals).
7. The lead foot should be pointed forward. Now turn the trailing foot out to about 45°. The feet should not be "tight-roping;" the front heel should be in line with the back heel so the back toes help balance.
8. Place the lead hand flat on the floor medial to (on the inside of) the lead foot.

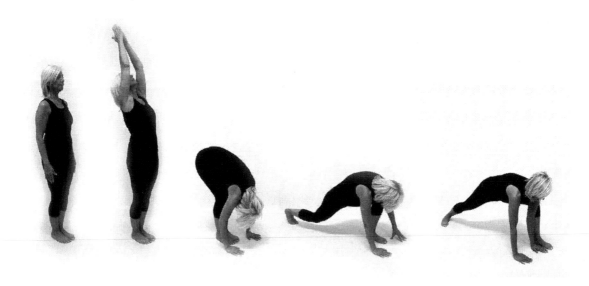

9. Raise the arm of the trailing side above the head and continue over the head until it is at about a 30° angle to the floor. The trailing leg, the torso, and the trailing side arm should approximate a straight line that sits at about a 30° angle to the floor.

10. Use the leading side's shoulder to push against the inside of the lead knee to keep the lead shin vertical and help place the lead shoulder directly under the trailing side's shoulder.

11. Pull the hips under the torso. When viewed from above, the body, from foot to hand, should be in a straight line.

12. Ensure that the lumbar, thoracic, and cervical vertebrae are in normal extension and then turn the head to look up at the trailing side inner elbow or the ceiling.

13. Hold for five breath cycles.

14. Return to the forward fold position (reverse the process until the feet are together and both hands on the floor) then repeat the sequence on the opposite side.

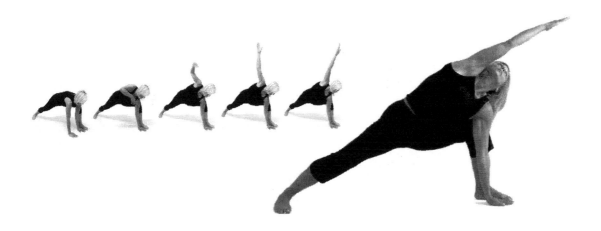

What are the benefits?

1. Improves balance, coordination, and posture.
2. Improves range of motion through stretching of the hips (adductors - adductor brevis, adductor longus, adductor magnus, pectineus, and gracilis; extensors - semitendinosus, semimembranosus, and biceps femoris), back (latissimus dorsi, quadratus lumborum), lateral abdomen (externus obliquus, internus obliquus), and lateral thorax (intercostalis, serratus anterior).
3. For beginners, provides a strength stimulus for the quadriceps (rectus femoris, vastus medialis, vastus lateralis, vastus intermedus) and gluteals.
4. When included as a part of a training sequence, this posture aids in the reduction of anxiety, depression, and perceived stress.
5. Develops local muscular endurance in all muscles actively contracting in the posture.

Contraindications

While this is a somewhat difficult posture to attain correctly, it is a low risk movement. There is no orthostatic challenge and only a minor increase in non-contraction induced resistance to blood flow (one arm overhead). Individuals with diagnosed hip, knee, or neck pathologies may require modification or may wish to not participate in the posture.

Learning and Teaching Checklist

1. Are the trainee's feet spread widely apart forward to back? ◯
2. Is the lead leg bent at 90° at the knee? ◯
3. Is the trailing leg straight with the foot flat on the floor and pointed laterally? ◯
4. Do the trailing leg, torso, and overhead arm form a 30° straight line to the floor? ◯
5. Are the leading ankle, knee, and both shoulders stacked in a vertical line? ◯
6. Is the trainee breathing throughout? ◯
7. Does the trainee hold the final position for five full breath cycles? ◯

Rotated Side Angle ~ Parivrtta Parsvakonasana ~

This is an intense and difficult twisting posture that improves mobility of the vertebral column and the hip. It is the slightly more complicated cousin of the Extended Side Angle.

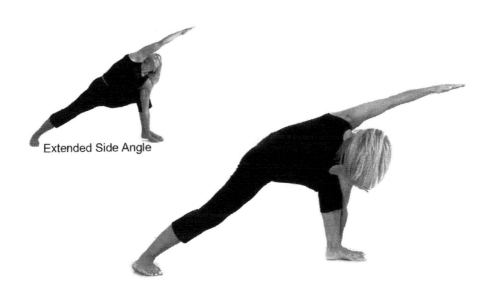

Extended Side Angle

Note how the torso orientation differs from the Extended Side Angle.

How to do it

1. Begin in Mountain posture.
2. Raise the hands above the head, elbows extended as much as possible, biceps facing the ears, and palms together if possible.
3. Bend forward into Forward Fold (refer to description in Triplet 1).
4. Look up and extend the spine, hands flat on the floor.
5. Step back with one foot, keep the lead knee at 90° and knee in line with the ankle. Rest hands palms flat on either side of the front leg to keep balance during foot placement.

6. For beginners the feet should be far enough apart to feel a mild stretch in the thighs. For experienced trainees the feet should be spaced about 1½ leg lengths apart (this could be more than 4 feet in long legged individuals).

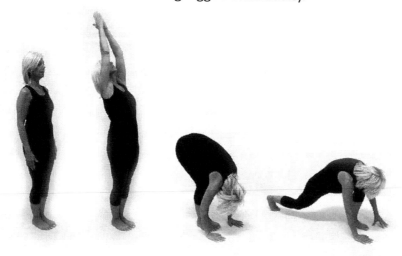

7. The lead foot should be pointed forward. Now turn the trailing foot out to about 45°. The feet should not be "tight-roping;" the front heel should be in line with the back heel so the back toes help balance.
8. Place the hands flat on the lead knee then bring the torso upright, pushing into the knee with the palm.
9. Gently pull the knee toward and over the mid line of the body then lower the torso toward the lead leg. Reach the trailing-side arm diagonally over the knee, bending the elbow, then rest the elbow as far down the outer (lateral) side of the lead shin as possible, then place the hand flat on the floor lateral to the foot.
10. Use the trailing side's arm as a lever to twist the torso around and to place the shoulders directly under each other.
11. Extend the lead side's arm forward and upward.
12. Bring the shoulders down (depress the scapulae) and extend the neck as you turn the head to look up and over the shoulder.
13. Pull the hips under the torso. When viewed from above, the body, from foot to hand, should roughly be in a straight line.
14. Ensure that the lumbar, thoracic, and cervical vertebrae are in normal extension and then turn the head to look up at the trailing-side inner elbow or the ceiling.

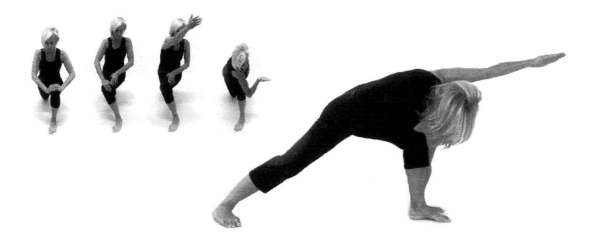

15. Hold for five breath cycles.
16. To change sides, unwind from the posture and move the body to the opposite end of the mat and into the lunge position. Repeat the sequence on the opposite side.

What are the benefits?

1. Improves balance, coordination, and posture.
2. Improves range of motion through stretching of the hips (adductors - adductor brevis, adductor longus, adductor magnus, pectineus, and gracilis; extensors - semitendinosus, semimembranosus, and biceps femoris), back (latissimus dorsi, quadratus lumborum), lateral abdomen (externus obliquus, internus obliquus), and lateral thorax (intercostalis, serratus anterior).
3. For beginners, provides a strength stimulus for the quadriceps (rectus femoris, vastus medialis, vastus lateralis, vastus intermedus) and gluteals.
4. When included as a part of a training sequence, this posture aids in the reduction of anxiety, depression, and perceived stress.
5. Develops local muscular endurance in all muscles actively contracting in the posture.

Contraindications

This is a difficult posture to attain correctly and there are substantial torsional forces in place on the vertebral column. Individuals with diagnosed knee, hip, back, or neck pathologies may require modification or may wish to not participate in the posture.

There is no orthostatic challenge and only a minor increase in non-contraction induced resistance to blood flow (one arm overhead).

Learning and Teaching Checklist

1. Are the feet spread widely apart? ○
2. Is the leading leg bent approximately 90° at the knee? ○
3. Is the trailing leg straight with the foot flat on the floor? ○
4. Is the torso rotated? ○
5. Do the trailing leg, torso, and overhead arm form a straight line at about 30° to the floor? ○
6. Are the leading ankle, knee, and both shoulders stacked in a vertical line? ○
7. Is the head turned and gaze directed upwards? ○
8. Is the trainee breathing throughout? ○
9. Does the trainee hold the final position for five full breath cycles? ○

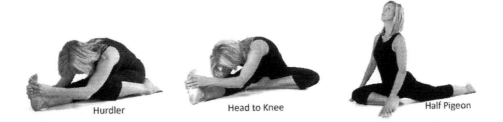

Hurdler   Head to Knee   Half Pigeon

Hurdler   ~ Tiryan Mukhaikapada Pascimottanasana ~

This posture is commonly known as the "Hurdler's Stretch" as it approximates the position a track athlete assumes when clearing a hurdle. It or its close cousin, "Head to Knee," is used in virtually every stretching session conducted in amateur or professional sports. It is primarily used to develop mobility around the hip and knee.

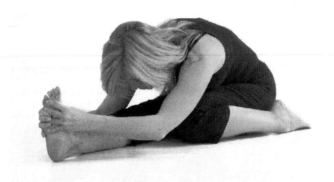

How to do it

1. Begin in an upright seated position. Later on we will formalize this position into a full posture (see Beginnings & Endings).

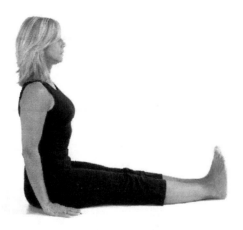

2. Lean to one side. This is now the lead side. Shift the bodyweight over onto the lead leg. Lift the trailing hip to fully shift your weight. Use the lead hand on the floor to assist in supporting weight and stability.

3. Bend the trailing knee up and lean it over the lead leg (flex the knee, adduct the hip). This will leave the trailing foot near to or still touching the floor.

4. Hold the trailing ankle with the trailing hand and gently pull the trailing shin and calf back until they form a line with the ankle just lateral to the hip. It is imperative here to keep the lower leg tight against the thigh in order to limit stress on the knee.

5. Both ischial tuberosities should be on the floor, but some individuals with well-developed muscle mass may find it difficult to get both butt bones, the bent knee, shin, and ankle on the floor at the same time. This is not due to poor flexibility, but to anatomical hindrance (anatomy's version of chemistry's steric hindrance). Regardless, try to get the hips as level as possible. A block can be used under the lower hip for stability and balance.

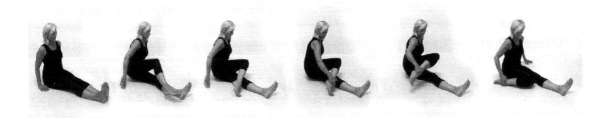

6. Keep the lead leg straight with the toes pointed up. Some individuals will not be able to fully extend the knee. Strategies to help with knee extension are to point the toes down (plantar flexion) or look up (cervical extension). Both of these reduce muscular tension along the posterior kinetic chain.

7. Engage the abdominal musculature. You should feel like you are attempting to pull your navel back towards the vertebral column. Place the hands outside of the thighs.

8. Keeping the vertebral column in normal extension, slowly lean forward through flexion of the hips and move to the hips' full range of motion. The hands should move down the legs as the torso leans toward the extended foot. The foot should be held, if possible, by grasping around the mid-foot.

9. Once the limit of range of motion of the hip is reached (sensed through hamstring discomfort), exhale and slowly pull the chest closer to the thigh. The result should be the abdomen and chest coming in contact with the thigh while keeping the entire vertebral column in normal extension.
10. The hands should end with the thumbs on top of the foot and the fingers wrapped around the bottom. Many people will be unable to assume this position initially so a strap can be used or they can hold near the ankles.
11. Keep the neck in normal extension. If there is separation between the chest and leg (beginners or those with poor flexibility), keep the eyes slightly forward rather than tucking the chin down and back.

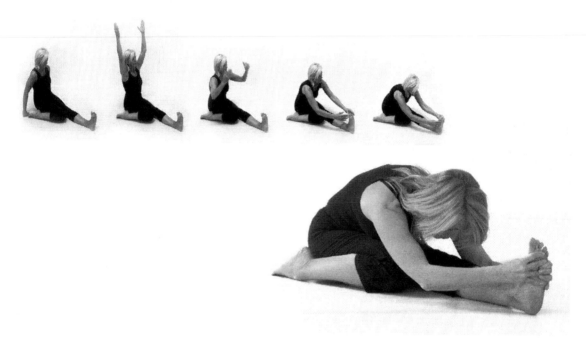

12. Hold for five breath cycles.
13. Return to the seated upright posture and repeat the above sequence on the opposite side.

What are the benefits?

1. Improves hip and lower back range of motion through longitudinal stretching of the hamstrings (semitendinosus, semimembranosus, biceps femoris), gluteals, quadratus lumborum, and erectors spinae.

2. Improves knee range of motion through stretching of quadriceps (vastus lateralis, vastus medialis, vastus internus, and rectus femoris).
3. Improves sitting and standing posture.
4. When included as a part of a training sequence, this posture aids in the reduction of anxiety, depression, and perceived stress.
5. Develops local muscular endurance in all muscles actively contracting in the posture.

Contraindications

Individuals with diagnosed low back, hip or knee problems may wish to abstain from this posture or to use a modification. Later term pregnancy will prevent participation in this posture.

Learning and Teaching Checklist

1. Are the ischial tuberosities on the floor (or one elevated on a block if needed)? ◯
2. Is the leading leg completely extended with toes up? ◯
3. Is the trailing leg straight: flexed tightly at the knee – shin, knee, and ankle on the floor? ◯
4. Is the torso flexed forward at the hip and making contact with the thigh? ◯
5. Is the vertebral column held in a close approximation of normal extension? ◯
6. Are the arms extended forward with fingers around the ball of the feet? ◯
7. Is the neck in normal extension? ◯
8. Is the trainee breathing throughout? ◯
9. Does the trainee hold the final position for five full breath cycles? ◯

Head to Knee   ~ Janu Sirsasana ~

This seated posture aids in developing range of motion around the hips, through posterior and medial stretching. The name "Head to Knee" can be somewhat misleading as individuals with abnormally long or short vertebral columns and/or femurs will only be able to approximate the head-knee relationship. For this reason, "Chest to Thigh" also works as an anatomical descriptor for this posture.

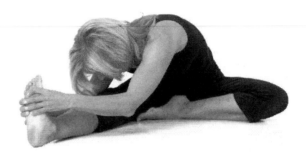

How to do it

1. Begin in an upright seated posture.

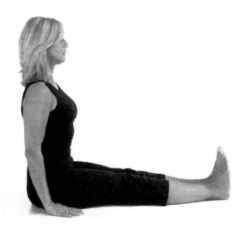

2. Rotate one leg out until the knee and toes point out to the side (laterally). This is the now the trailing side. Keep the opposite knee extended and the toes pointed upwards. This is now the lead side.

3. Bend the trailing knee and pull the trailing heel to a level above the lead knee. Place the sole of the trailing foot flat along the inside of the lead leg. The toes of the trailing foot will point down towards the foot of the lead leg. In beginners and those with poor flexibility the trailing knee may be slightly up in the air and not resting on the floor. This is fine; gravity will provide a gentle and natural stretch that will aid in increasing lateral mobility at the hip over time.

4. Slightly rotate the torso so the lead leg is perpendicular to the line from shoulder to shoulder. Place the hands on top of the lead thigh.

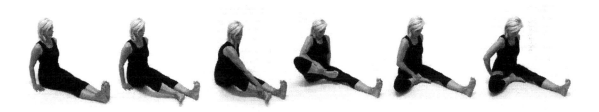

5. Lift the arms above the head and stretch the fingers toward the ceiling. Engage the abdominal musculature to pull the anterior wall towards the vertebral column. Sit tall and reach up to create a feeling of torso length and height.

6. Slowly lean forward at the hips until they are at the limit of their range of motion. Only then begin slowly allowing the lumbar vertebrae to flex forward, thus bringing the chest closer to the thigh.

7. Reach as far forward as possible and wrap both hands around the bottom of the balls of the foot of the extended leg. To accomplish this, the thoracic vertebrae may need to be flexed forward. If the feet cannot be reached, the ankle can be grasped or a strap can be looped under the foot. Gently pull the torso forward to create a stretch.

8. Keep the neck in normal extension. If there is separation between the chest and leg (in beginners or those with poor flexibility), gently extend the neck and tilt the head up.

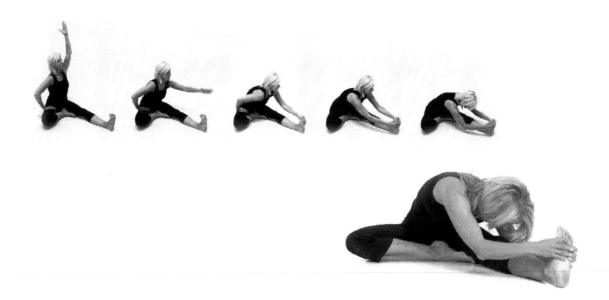

9. Hold for five breath cycles.
10. Return to the seated upright posture and repeat the above on the opposite side.

What are the benefits?

1. Improves hip and lower back range of motion through longitudinal stretching of the hamstrings (semitendinosus, semimembranosus, biceps femoris), gluteals, quadratus lumborum, erectors spinae, and through lateral stretching of the adductors (adductor brevis, adductor longus, adductor magnus, pectineus, gracilis).
2. Improves sitting and standing posture.
3. When included as a part of a training sequence, this posture aids in the reduction of anxiety, depression, and perceived stress.
4. Develops local muscular endurance in all muscles actively contracting in the posture.

Contraindications

Individuals with diagnosed low back, hip, or knee problems may wish to abstain from this posture or to use a modification.

Learning and Teaching Checklist

1. Are the ischial tuberosities on the floor?   ◯
2. Is the leading leg completely extended with toes up?   ◯

3. Is the sole of one foot on the inner thigh of the opposite leg, knees bent, toes forward? ○

4. Is the torso flexed forward at the hip and making contact with the leading thigh? ○

5. Is the vertebral column held in a close approximation of normal extension? ○

6. Are the arms extended forward with fingers around the ball of the feet? ○

7. Is the neck in normal extension? ○

8. Is the trainee breathing throughout? ○

9. Does the trainee hold the final position for five full breath cycles? ○

Half Pigeon   ~ Eka Pada Kapotasana ~

The Half Pigeon is a partially seated posture that strongly develops range of motion around the hip in flexion, extension, and lateral rotation.

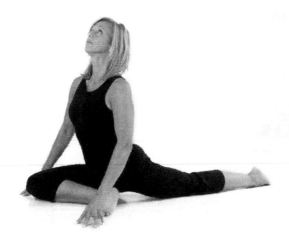

How to do it

1. Start in Down Dog position.

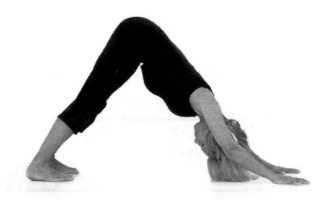

2. Come up on your toes. Turn (externally rotate) one knee out. The side on which you choose to rotate the knee outward is now the lead side (in the following illustrations, the lead side is the left).

3. Lift the lead foot and step forward. The lead foot should touch down six inches behind the trailing hand. The toes should be pointing directly forward.

4. Lay the shin down across the width of the mat.

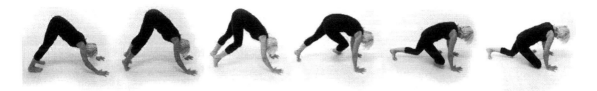

5. Sink the hips back towards the floor by extending (straightening) the trailing knee along the mat, straight to the rear. At the same time the lead hip should be relaxed into flexion. This will place the lateral aspect of the lead thigh on the floor.
6. Extend the back to attain an upright position with vertebrae held in normal lordotic and kyphotic extension. The cervical vertebrae should be in slight extension with an upward gaze. The scapulae are depressed (pull them toward the buttocks).
7. The hands should be at the front of the lead knee and lead foot. The fingertips should make light contact with the floor.
8. Push the trailing hip down towards the lead ankle and floor. Use gravity and muscle contraction (iliacus and psoas) to pull the hips into line.

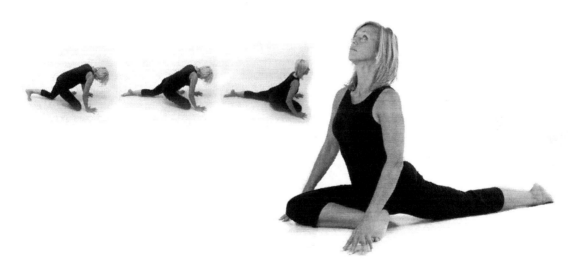

9. Hold for five breath cycles.
10. Reverse the movements to return to Down Dog position.
11. Perform the posture with the opposite side.

What are the benefits?

1. Improves hip and lower back range of motion through longitudinal stretching of the hamstrings (semitendinosus, semimembranosus, biceps femoris) of the lead leg, and the rectus femoris and sartorius of the trailing leg. It also places a rotational stretch on the the hip via the adductors (adductor brevis, adductor longus, adductor magnus, pectineus, gracilis) and the hip's rotator cuff (piriformis, gemelli, and obturator internus).
2. Helps develop motor control of the lower back musculature.
3. Improves sitting and standing posture.
4. When included as a part of a training sequence, this posture aids in the reduction of anxiety, depression, and perceived stress.
5. Develops local muscular endurance in all muscles actively contracting in the posture.

Contraindications

Individuals with diagnosed low back, hip or knee problems may wish to abstain from this posture or to use a modification.

Learning and Teaching Checklist

1. Is the lead leg flexed forward at the hip and in lateral rotation, shin across the body? ◯
2. Is the leading leg buttocks seated on the floor? ◯
3. Is the trailing leg fully extended to the rear, with thigh, shin, and top of foot on floor? ◯
4. Is the torso held in normal extension (not supported on arms)? ◯
5. Are the hands (fingertips) placed on the floor just lateral to the lead knee and foot? ◯
6. Is the chest up and the shoulders retracted to the rear? ◯
7. Cervical vertebrae in slight extension, head tilted upward slightly? ◯
8. Is the trainee breathing throughout? ◯
9. Does the trainee hold the final position for five full breath cycles? ◯

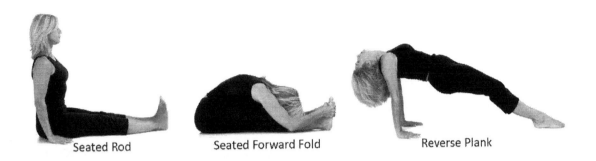

Seated Rod   Seated Forward Fold   Reverse Plank

Seated Rod

~ Dandasana ~

This posture is a mild low back, hip, and knee stretch but is more useful as a means of reinforcing correct posture. It is a simple sitting posture and will serve as a starting point or transition for all seated postures.

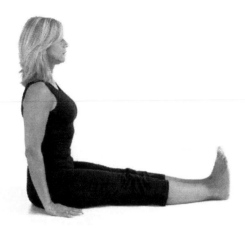

How to do it

1. Begin by sitting on the floor, legs straight in front of the body and together. You may need to internally rotate the legs (roll them towards the middle) to get the feet together.
2. Dorsiflex the ankles (point the toes straight up). Keep pulling the toes up towards the torso until the heels elevate slightly from the floor. This stretches the calf musculature. By gently contracting the quadriceps, a small stretch will be placed on the hamstrings.

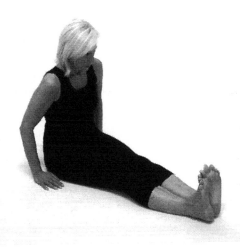

3. Pull the torso forward until it forms a 90° angle with the legs (and floor).
4. Lift the chest by arching the low back and pulling the shoulders back to create normal extension of the lumbar and thoracic vertebrae. This upper body orientation is much like that of military "attention" position. By doing this correctly, the ischial tuberosities (butt bones) will be firmly anchored on the floor.
5. The cervical vertebrae should be in normal extension and the head and gaze should be directed straight forward. The spine may feel straight, like a rod or staff, but the curve of the spine will still be present.
6. The arms should be directly by the sides of the body with the hands flat on the floor directly under the shoulders, fingers pointed forward. Extend the elbows.

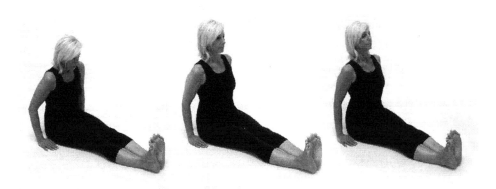

What are the benefits?

1. Improves standing and sitting posture.
2. Improves hip flexibility by stretching the hamstrings (semitendinosus, semimembranosus, biceps femoris) and gastrocnemius.
3. In beginners, improves strength of back extensors (erector spinae, latissimus dorsi, trapezius), hip flexors (sartorius, rectus femoris), and lumbar flexors (iliacus, psoas).
4. When included as a part of a training sequence, this posture aids in the reduction of anxiety, depression, and perceived stress.
5. Develops local muscular endurance in all muscles actively contracting in the posture.

Contraindications

None.

Learning and Teaching Checklist

1. Is the weight even on the hips and are the ischial tuberosities on the floor? ○
2. Are the legs together and knees fully extended in front of the body? ○
3. Are the feet together, ankles in normal flexion (toes pointed up)? ○
4. Is the hip angle at 90°? ○
5. Are the lumbar, thoracic, and cervical vertebrae held in normal extension (no slouching)? ○
6. Are the head and gaze straight forward? ○
7. Are the arms to the side with hands on the floor directly under the shoulders? ○
8. Are the fingers pointed straight forward? ○
9. Is the trainee breathing throughout? ○
10. Does the trainee hold the final position for five full breath cycles? ○

Seated Forward Fold   ~ Pachimottonasana ~

What is the pose?

This is a seated, aggressive hamstring stretch that improves mobility of the hips and low back.

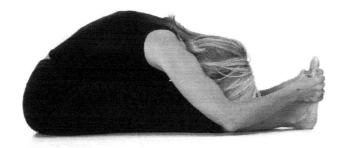

How to do it

1. Begin in the Seated Rod posture.

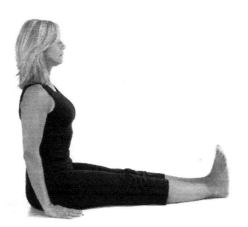

2. Raise the arms laterally from both sides of the body. Rotate the arms at the shoulder so the palms face each other. Sit erect. Engage the abdominal musculature (you should feel like you are attempting to pull your navel back towards the vertebral column). Tilt the hips forward to firmly seat the ischial tuberosities on the floor.

3. Maintain arm direction and move the arms toward the feet by leaning the torso slowly forward. This movement occurs only at the hips, not by rounding the back.

4. Maintain normal extension or a flat lower back for as long as possible. As the abdomen comes into contact with the upper thighs there will be some inevitable rounding of the lumbar and thoracic vertebrae. The goal is to minimize this as much as possible. Engaging the abdominal musculature to pull the anterior wall towards the vertebral column will aid in this effort.

5. Reach as far forward with the hands as possible. Reach over the top of the foot and wrap the first two fingers around the big toes. Beginners and those with poor flexibility will need to grab the side and back of the ankles or shins. Those with more range of motion can grab around the soles of the feet. Bending the knees slightly can help those with poor flexibility. Once the grip is achieved, engage the quadriceps to produce a controlled hamstring stretch.

6. Look just over the toes while keeping the chin slightly tucked in towards the chest (this will keep the cervical vertebrae in normal extension). Do not drop the head to look down. Sit tall with the torso as you pull gently forward and down. Move the torso tighter and tighter to the top of the thighs with each subsequent breath.

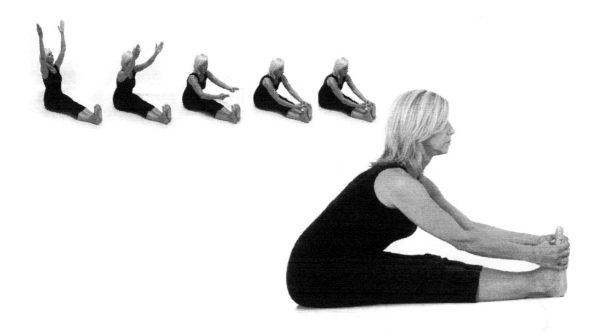

7. Gently allow the back to round as you pull forward to create a stretch along the back.

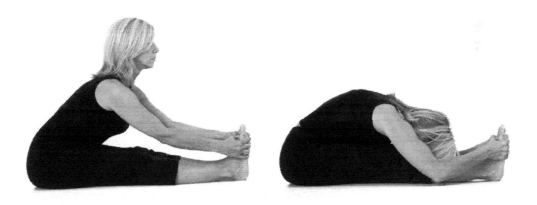

8. Hold for five breath cycles.

What are the benefits?

1. Improves hip and lower back range of motion through stretching the hamstrings (semitendinosus, semimembranosus, biceps femoris), gluteals, quadratus lumborum, erectors spinae, and to a small degree the latissimus dorsi.
2. Improves sitting posture.
3. When included as a part of a training sequence, this posture aids in the reduction of anxiety, depression, and perceived stress.
4. Develops local muscular endurance in all muscles actively contracting in the posture.

Contraindications

Those with diagnosed hip and low back problems may need to avoid participating in the posture.

Learning and Teaching Checklist

1. Are the ischial tuberosities on the floor and weight distributed evenly left to right? ○
2. Are both knees extended fully in front of the body, with legs and feet together? ○ ○
3. Is the torso leaning forward with back held in normal extension through early movement? ○
4. Torso contacting the thighs in the later movement (or moving closer with each breath)? ○
5. Is the movement mostly from the hip with no excessive lumbar and thoracic rounding? ○
6. Arms extended with fingers around the big toes (or around the ankles or balls of the feet)? ○
7. Is the head facing forward towards the toes? ○
8. Is the trainee breathing throughout? ○
9. Does the trainee hold the final position for five full breath cycles? ○

Reverse Plank   ~ Purvotanasana ~

This is a static body hold that develops midline stability along the posterior side of the body and improves mobility around the shoulder.

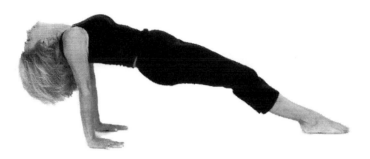

How to do it

1. Begin in the Seated Rod posture.

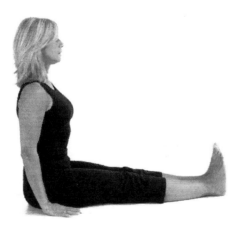

2. Move your hands to where the fingertips are approximately six inches behind the buttocks.

3. Slightly bend the knees and slide the feet a few inches closer to the buttocks then push down into the palms by extending the elbows, depressing the scapulae, lifting the chest up and forward, and rolling the head slightly back.
4. Lift the hips slightly off the floor and rest the body weight on the palms and heels of the feet.

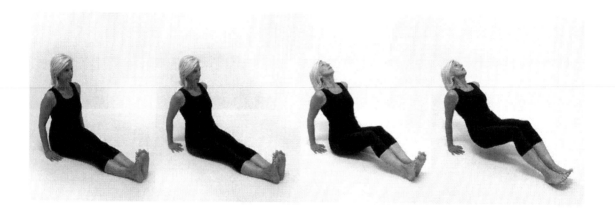

5. Lift the hips higher toward the ceiling. Point the toes down and flatten the soles of the feet on the floor (plantar flexion). The ankles and knees should be held together throughout the posture. For beginners it may not be possible to support bodyweight on the hands and arms. Bending the knees slightly to a point where the feet can be placed flat on the floor is an appropriate modification.
6. Push the feet down against the floor and push the hips up towards the ceiling. Gently roll the head back, extending the neck, lift the chest, and pull the shoulders down and toward the midline.
7. In the final position, the arms should be vertical. The shoulders, hips, knees and ankles should approximate a straight line slanting down from the shoulders to the floor.

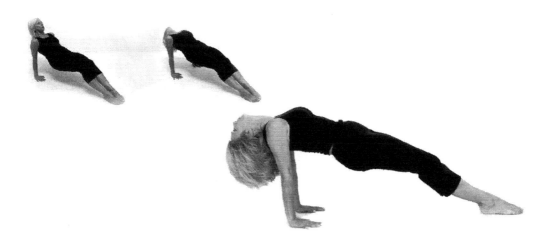

8. Hold for five breath cycles.

What are the benefits?

1. Improves midline stability by developing control of the hamstrings (semitendinosus, semimembranosus, biceps femoris), gluteals, erectors spinae, quadratus lumborum, latissimus dorsi, trapezius, rhomboideus, posterior deltoids, triceps brachii, and anterior neck musculature (sternoceidomastoid, scalenus). In beginners, strength is developed in all of these muscles.
2. Develops range of motion around the anterior shoulder by placing a stretch on the anterior deltoids, and pectoralis major.
3. Improves standing posture.
4. When included as a part of a training sequence, this posture aids in the reduction of anxiety, depression, and perceived stress.
5. Develops local muscular endurance in all muscles actively contracting in the posture.

Contraindications

Individuals with diagnosed wrist or low back problems may wish to avoid participation in this posture.

Learning and Teaching Checklist

1. Are the hands at the rear of the hips and knees slightly bent during set up? ◯
2. Are the feet flat on the floor and together? ◯
3. Are the knees extended and together? ◯
4. Are the shoulders, hips, knees, and ankles in line when viewed in profile? ◯
5. Is the chest up, shoulders back and down, neck extended? ◯
6. Are the arms vertical, hands directly under the shoulders and flat on the floor, and the fingertips pointed towards the feet? ◯
7. Cervical vertebrae in extension, chin pointed towards the ceiling? ◯
8. Is the trainee breathing throughout? ◯
9. Does the trainee hold the final position for five full breath cycles? ◯

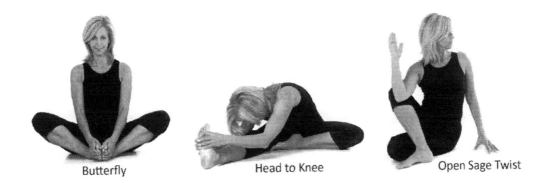

Butterfly   Head to Knee   Open Sage Twist

Butterfly ~ Baddhakonasana ~

This is an effective seated groin stretch that is used ubiquitously throughout athletics.

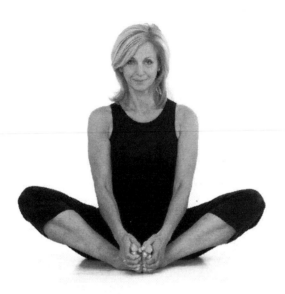

How to do it

1. Begin in the Seated Rod posture.

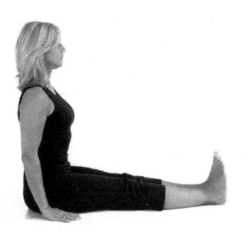

2. Bend and lift one knee (now the lead) off the floor (flex the knee and hip). As the thigh moves closer to the torso, abduct the hip and let gravity pull the knee out to the side. At the same time pull the heel in close to the groin.

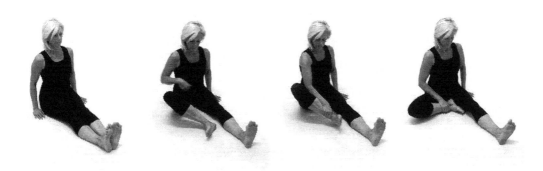

3. Repeat the same sequence with the opposite leg. Place the medial edges of the feet tightly together. Keep the torso fully erect.
4. Abduct the thighs (use the lateral thigh musculature to pull the knees down and laterally towards the floor). The soles of the feet should come into contact with each other.

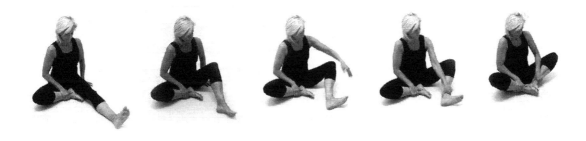

5. Bring your hands behind the buttocks, hand making a fist. Push down to slightly lift the buttocks off the floor. Use friction to keep the feet and calves in position and bring the hips nearer the feet.

6. Sit the hips down, keep one hand behind the body for stability, then reach one hand down and wrap it around the foot.
7. Reach down and wrap the second hand around the other foot, the fingers around and under the lateral aspect and soles, the thumbs over the tops and arches. Ensure the arms are completely extended at the elbow.
8. Sit up vertically; reinforce the arch in the lumbar vertebrae. Keep the thoracic and cervical vertebrae in normal extension with the gaze directly forward. The ischial tuberosities should be firmly on the floor. Engage the abdominal musculature to pull the navel towards the vertebral column.
9. Squeeze the scapulae towards midline (retract) and lift the chest.

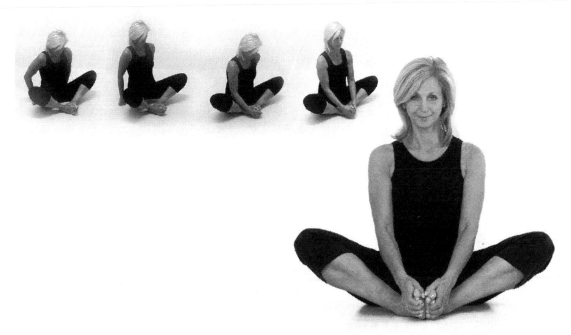

10. Hold for five breath cycles.

NOTE: It is the act of attaining complete normal vertebral extension relative to the pelvis that drives the stretch here. Erect posture and heels close to the crotch are the targets. It is common among sport practices to allow forward vertebral flexion (rounding of the back forward) in order to create a stretch by pulling up on the ankles and levering the elbows down on top of the knees. Such rounding reduces the overall effectiveness of the posture.

What are the benefits?

1. Provides a significant range of motion stimulus by stretching the adductors of the hip (adductor brevis, adductor magnus, adductor longus, pectineus), the iliacus, and the psoas.
2. Improves sitting and standing posture.
3. When included as a part of a training sequence, this posture aids in the reduction of anxiety, depression, and perceived stress.
4. Develops local muscular endurance in all muscles actively contracting in the posture.

Contraindications

This is a low risk posture requiring avoidance or modification only for those with diagnosed hip or groin problems.

Learning and Teaching Checklist

1. Ischial tuberosities in contact with the floor with weight symmetrically distributed? ◯
2. Are the soles of the feet together and the heels placed close to the groin? ◯
3. Hands wrapped around the feet with fingers under the foot and the thumbs over? ◯
4. Are the arms nearly straight but relaxed? ◯
5. Are the lumbar, thoracic and cervical vertebrae held in normal extension? ◯
6. Is the chest lifted and the shoulders back (scapulae retracted back)? ◯
7. Is the head up and gaze focused directly forward? ◯
8. Is the trainee breathing throughout? ◯
9. Does the trainee hold the final position for five full breath cycles? ◯

Head to Knee   ~ Janu Sirsasana ~

Refer to Triplet 5 for the full Head to Knee description.

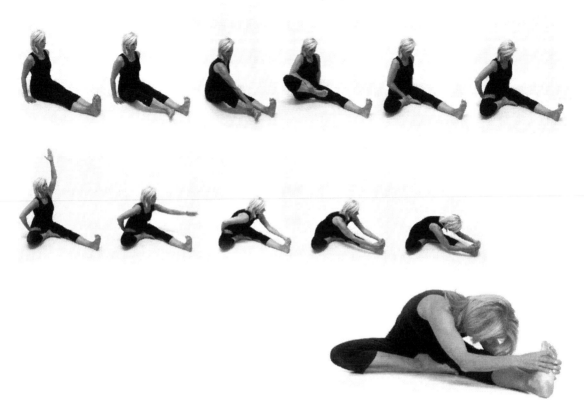

Make sure to hold the final position for five breath cycles.

Learning and Teaching Checklist

1. Are the ischial tuberosities on the floor (or one elevated on a block if needed)? ○
2. Is the leading leg completely extended with toes up? ○
3. Is the trailing leg straight: flexed tightly at the knee – shin, knee, and ankle on the floor? ○
4. Is the torso flexed forward at the hip and making contact with the thigh? ○
5. Is the vertebral column held in a close approximation of normal extension? ○
6. Are the arms extended forward with fingers around the ball of the feet? ○
7. Is the neck in normal extension? ○
8. Is the trainee breathing throughout? ○
9. Does the trainee hold the final position for five full breath cycles? ○

Open Sage Twist   ~ Marichyasana ~

This is a two-stage, seated, twisting posture that develops range of motion along the lumbar, thoracic, and cervical vertebrae. One arm pulls the shoulders around and the other arm uses leverage against one knee to stretch the entire vertebral column around its long axis. The arms, legs, and torso in this posture are oriented like those in the images of Egyptian tomb-art.

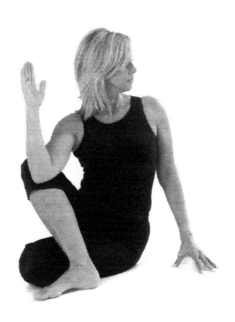

How to do it

1. Begin in the Seated Rod posture.

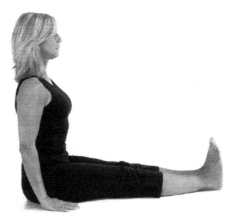

2. Place a hand at about mid-shin on the same-side leg. Slide this foot up and under the opposite leg. This is now the trailing leg (these illustrations use the right leg). The trailing heel should be in front of and just lateral to the opposite ischial tuberosity (or as close as possible). The trailing leg should be under the lead leg and the trailing foot on the outside of (lateral to) the bent lead leg.

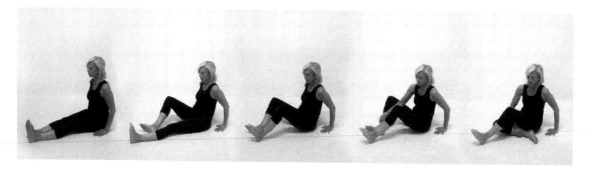

3. Grasp the lead shin about one third of the way up from the ankle and sweep the bent lead leg over the trailing thigh.
4. The lead foot should be placed flat on the floor near the trailing leg's thigh. The lead toes should only be slightly anterior to the trailing knee. Use both hands to adjust the position of both the right and left feet so they are tightly and firmly placed.

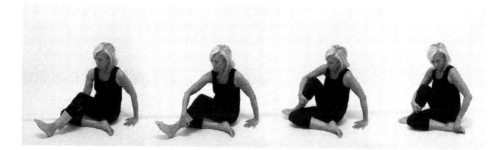

5. Sit firmly and evenly on the ischial tuberosities (butt bones). Sit tall with the vertebral column in normal extension (sit up, no slouching). Slowly and gently rotate the torso to the lead side (to the left in these illustrations).
6. Wrap the trailing arm around the lead knee and place the lead hand palm-down about six inches behind the lead hip to create torsion that pulls the shoulders into a line parallel to the legs. The fingers should be pointed directly away from and behind the body.

7. Keep the torso erect (normal lumbar, thoracic, and cervical extension) and look back over the lead shoulder. There should be a sensation of spiraling tension along the length of the spine.

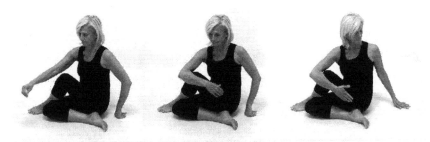

8. Hold for five breath cycles.
9. To change the direction of rotation, release the torsion on the shoulders, then place the lead elbow on the outside of the lead knee. Place the trailing arm and hand behind the trailing hip. Use the trailing arm and lead humerus (upper arm) to lever the shoulders (and vertebral column) into a larger degree of rotation.

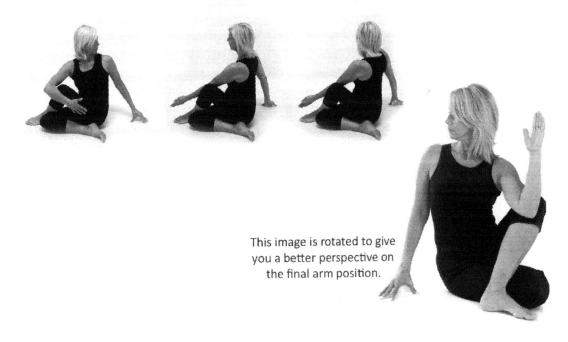

This image is rotated to give you a better perspective on the final arm position.

185

10. Hold for five breath cycles.
11. Return to the Seated Rod posture and repeat on the opposite side.

What are the benefits?

1. Improves rotational range of motion around the entire vertebral column (lumbar, thoracic, and cervical).
2. Can reduce the sensation of low back pain.
3. In beginners, increases the strength of the triceps brachii, posterior deltoids, and latissimus dorsi.
4. When included as a part of a training sequence, this posture aids in the reduction of anxiety, depression, and perceived stress.
5. Develops local muscular endurance in all muscles actively contracting in the posture.

Contraindications

Individuals with diagnosed low back problems should apply the stretch with caution, use a modification, or avoid participation.

Learning and Teaching Checklist

1. Are both ischial tuberosities on the floor? ◯
2. Is the knee of the trailing leg flexed, heel anterior and just lateral to the lead hip? ◯
3. Lead knee flexed, foot flat on the floor, toes lateral to and just in front of trailing knee? ◯
4. Is there full transitional rotation? ◯
5. Trailing arm placed about six inches behind the trailing hip, with fingertips on the floor? ◯
6. Lead arm with the elbow flexed placed on the medial side of the same side bent knee? ◯
7. Is the torso rotated so the shoulders are in a line parallel to the line of the legs? ◯
8. Head turned to the trailing side? ◯
9. Is the trainee breathing throughout? ◯
10. Does the trainee hold the final position for five full breath cycles? ◯

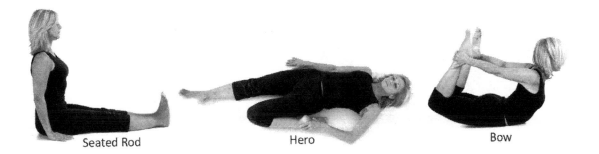

Seated Rod   Hero   Bow

Seated Rod

~ Dandasana ~

Refer to Triplet 6 for the full Seated Rod description.

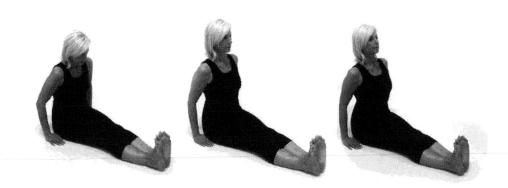

Make sure to hold the final position for five breath cycles.

Learning and Teaching Checklist

1. Is the weight even on the hips and are the ischial tuberosities on the floor? ◯
2. Are the legs together and knees fully extended in front of the body? ◯
3. Are the feet together, ankles in normal flexion (toes pointed up)? ◯
4. Is the hip angle at 90°? ◯
5. Are the lumbar, thoracic, and cervical vertebrae held in normal extension (no slouching)? ◯
6. Are the head and gaze straight forward? ◯
7. Are the arms to the side with hands on the floor directly under the shoulders? ◯
8. Are the fingers pointed straight forward? ◯
9. Is the trainee breathing throughout? ◯
10. Does the trainee hold the final position for five full breath cycles? ◯

Hero   ~ Virasana ~

This is a supine posture that creates a profound stretch around the knee and an anterior stretch on the ankles. As it places a stretch on the rectus femoris, it can also be felt on the front of the hip.

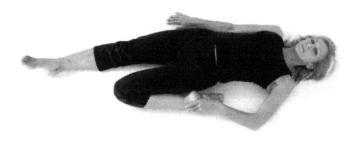

How to do it

1. Begin in the Seated Rod posture.

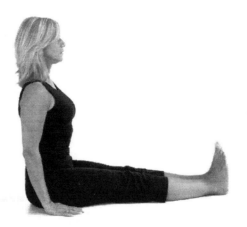

2. Lean to one side. This is now the lead side. Shift the bodyweight over onto the lead leg. Lift the trailing hip to fully shift your weight. Use the lead hand on the floor to assist in supporting weight and stability.

3. Bend the trailing knee up and lean it over the lead leg (flex the knee, adduct the hip). This will leave the trailing foot near to or still touching the floor.

4. Hold the trailing ankle with the trailing hand and gently pull the trailing shin and calf back until they form a line with the ankle just lateral to the hip. It is imperative here to keep the lower leg tight against the thigh in order to limit stress on the knee.

5. Both ischial tuberosities should be on the floor, but some individuals with well-developed muscle mass may find it difficult to get both butt bones, the bent knee, shin, and ankle on the floor at the same time. This is not due to poor flexibility, but to anatomical hindrance (anatomy's version of chemistry's steric hindrance). Regardless, try to get the hips as level as possible. A block can be used under the higher hip for stability and balance.

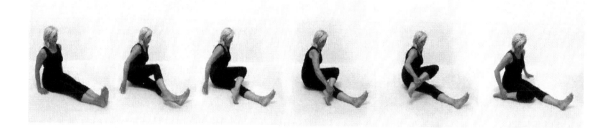

6. Once the butt bones touch the floor, ensure that the lumbar, thoracic, and cervical vertebrae are in normal extension. A common cue for this is to "sit tall" and is generally accomplished by lifting the chest, squeezing the scapulae together, and lifting the jawline.

7. Bend the elbow of the arm opposite the bent knee and carefully lower the body down until the elbow contacts the floor. For beginners, this may be as far as they are able to go in this posture.

8. If possible, lean back further and support the torso equally on the elbows. This is another intermediary position that can be used as a final posture if range of motion does not allow the next step.

9. Slowly lower the torso and place the back upon the floor. In the final posture the lumbar vertebrae should be in normal extension (no excessive arching).

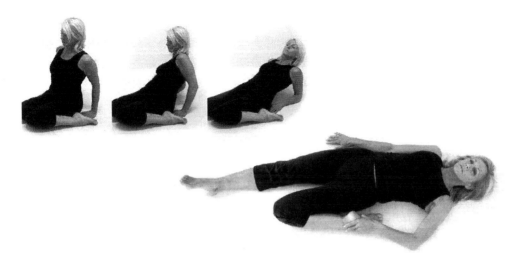

10. Hold for five breath cycles.

What are the benefits?

1. Improves knee range of motion through stretching of quadriceps (vastus lateralis, vastus medialis, vastus internus, and rectus femoris).
2. Improves anterior ankle range of motion (in plantar flexion) by placing a mild stretch on the anterior and lateral ankle musculature (tibialis anterior, extensor digitorum longus, extensor hallucis longus, fibularis longus).
3. Improves sitting and standing posture.
4. When included as a part of a training sequence, this posture aids in the reduction of anxiety, depression, and perceived stress.
5. Develops local muscular endurance in all muscles actively contracting in the posture.

Contraindications

This is a low risk posture; however, individuals with diagnosed knee problems may wish to avoid or modify this posture.

Learning and Teaching Checklist

1. One knee flexed with shins, ankles, top of feet, and toes parallel and contacting the floor?   ◯

2. One knee extended forward with toes upward?   ◯

3. Are the hips level with ischial tuberosities on the floor (a block used as needed)?   ◯

4. Backwards torso lean used appropriately to place back on or in proximity to the floor?   ◯

5. Is the line of the shoulders parallel to the floor?   ◯

6. Are the lumbar, thoracic, and cervical vertebrae in normal extension?   ◯

7. Are the arms comfortably placed with palms down (pronated) on the extended leg side and on the foot of the bent leg side?   ◯

8. Is the trainee breathing throughout?   ◯

9. Does the trainee hold the final position for five full breath cycles?   ◯

Bow   ~ Dhanurasana ~

This challenging posture provides a significant anterior body stretch and develops posterior range of motion at the shoulder. As it requires a degree of isometric muscular contraction to assume the posture, local muscular endurance is also improved.

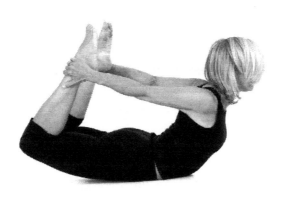

How to do it

1. Lie face down on the floor with the feet separated slightly.
2. Place the hands on the floor directly under the shoulder joints.
3. While keeping the feet touching the floor, elevate the hands and chest off of the floor. This is often called the "Superman" position.
4. Once the chest is up, raise the feet off the floor (keep the knees straight). Relax back into the original position. This prepares joints and musculature to move into the full posture.

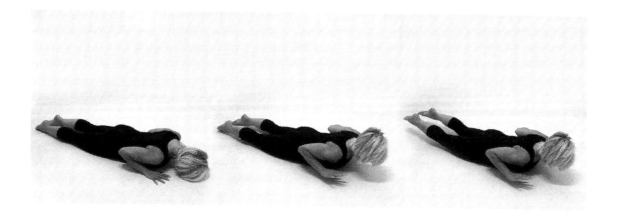

5. Move the feet slightly wider to approximately hip width.
6. Bend (flex) one knee and bring the foot as close to the buttocks as possible.
7. Reach back with the same side hand and grasp around the ankle (lateral to anterior).
8. Flex the opposite knee and bring the foot as close to the buttocks as possible.
9. Reach back with the same side hand and grasp around the ankle. Note that the wider the knees, the easier it is to grab the ankles but once the ankles are in hand the knees must be moved back to hip width.

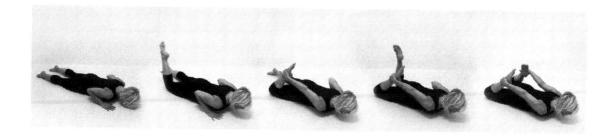

10. Inhale and push the ankles into the hands. Lift the chest and head and then lift the knees off of the floor.
11. Point the toes (plantar flex the foot).
12. Actively engage the lumbar musculature to arch the low back and tense the abdominal musculature.
13. Slightly extend the cervical vertebrae (tilt the head back slightly) to gaze forward and slightly upward. Hold for a few seconds then exhale and release.

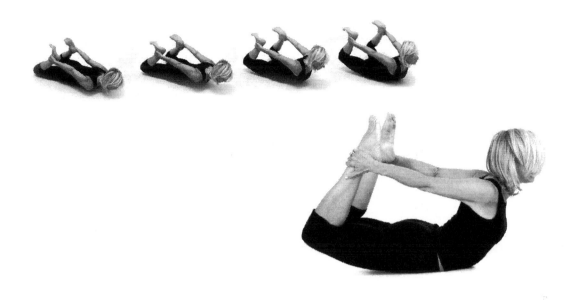

14. Repeat for five breath cycles. Extend the duration of the hold with each repeat if possible. If you can't reach the feet, a strap can be used around the ankles and held with each hand, arms extended.

What are the benefits?

1. Provides a significant anterior shoulder range of motion stimulus through stretching the anterior deltoideus, pectoralis major and pectoralis minor.
2. Increases lumbar vertebral range of motion by placing an anterior stretch on the rectus abdominis and through recruitment of lumbar vertebral extensors (erectors spinae, quadratus lumborum).
3. Ankle mobility (ability to fully plantar flex the ankle) is developed through the tension and stretch provided by the hands grasping the ankle and proximal metatarsals (stretches the tibialis anterior and extensor digitorum longus).
4. When included as a part of a training sequence, this posture aids in the reduction of anxiety, depression, and perceived stress.
5. Develops local muscular endurance in all muscles actively contracting in the posture.

Contraindications

Individuals with diagnosed shoulder or lumbar vertebral problems may wish to avoid participation or use a modification. Pregnancy is a definitive contraindication.

Learning and Teaching Checklist

1. Is the preparatory elevation of the chest and legs accomplished? ○
2. Is the ankle grasped correctly? ○
3. In the final position are the hips and abdomen supporting the bodyweight? ○
4. Are the knees at hip width and elevated off the floor? ○
5. Are the arms extended backwards with the elbows extended? ○
6. Are the hands grasping the ankles in correct position with the thumbs down? ○
7. Is the chest up? ○
8. Is the head tilted up slightly? ○
9. Is the trainee breathing throughout? ○
10. Does the trainee hold the final position for five full breath cycles? ○

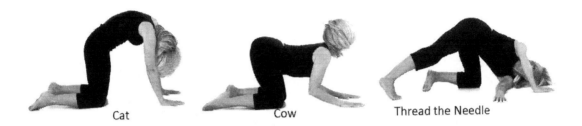

Cat Cow Thread the Needle

Cat   ~ Marjaryasana ~

What is the pose?

This is a simple hands-and-knees posture that uses hip, abdominal, and pectoral muscle contraction to drive a stretch along the posterior shoulder and the lumbar and thoracic vertebrae. The name comes from the rounded-back stretch cats commonly engage in. A crude parallel is the position that intoxicated people often assume as they pray to the porcelain god after a hard night out.

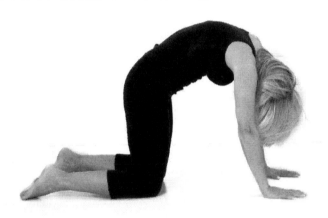

How to do it

1. Start in a kneeling position with the knees directly under the shoulders. The hips should be fully extended. The shins, tops of the feet, and toes should be in contact with the floor and point directly back (parallel to each other and perpendicular to the line of the shoulders).
2. Bend forward at the hips (flexion) and place the hands flat on the floor, fingers pointed directly forward. Slide the hands forward until both the arms and thighs are perpendicular to the floor.

3. In this intermediary "tabletop" position, the complete vertebral column should be in normal extension.

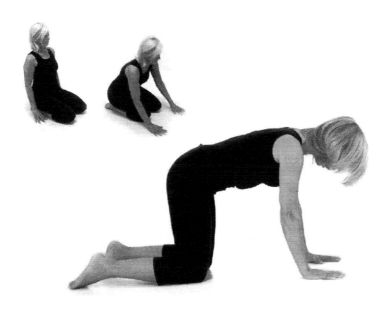

4. Execute a slow, powerful exhalation and contract the abdominal muscles. Try to pull the pelvis up and the rib cage down towards the navel. Forcefully contract the chest musculature to pull the shoulders towards midline.
5. Roll the head forward with the chin tucked in to flex the cervical spine. Ensure that the complete vertebral column, tailbone to base of skull, is in flexion.
6. Return to the tabletop position by moving into normal extension of the vertebral column.
7. Repeat this sequence for five cycles..

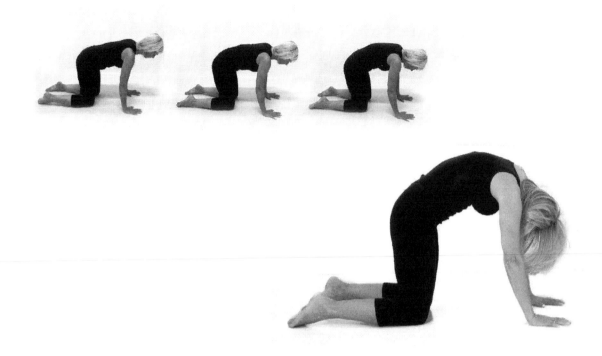

NOTE: After learning the Cat posture and the subsequent Cow posture, there is a direct transition from one to the other. The positions directly alternate through the Table posture without hesitation and without returning to the kneeling position.

What are the benefits?

1. A primary benefit is development of vertebral (lumbar and thoracic) range of motion through stretching of the vertebral extensors (erectors spinae, multifidus, quadratus lumborum, intertransversarii, rotatores).
2. Another primary benefit is development of shoulder range of motion through stretching of the posterior shoulder and back musculature (trapezius, latissimus dorsi, rhomboideus, levator scapulae, posterior deltoideus).
3. In beginners, strength will be developed in the contracting anterior musculature.
4. When included as a part of a training sequence, this posture aids in the reduction of anxiety, depression, and perceived stress.

5. Develops local muscular endurance in all muscles actively contracting in the posture.

Contraindications

This is an extremely low risk posture. Individuals with diagnosed vertebral problems may want to avoid the posture or modify the degree of vertebral flexion.

Learning and Teaching Checklist

1. Has the table top starting position been assumed correctly?   ○
2. Knees at approximate shoulder width?   ○
3. Knees, shins, ankles, tops of feet, and toes on the floor?   ○
4. Knee angle approximately 90°?   ○
5. Lumbar and thoracic back rounded/in significant anterior flexion?   ○
6. Shoulders rounded side-to-side when viewed from the front of the posture?   ○
7. Arms perpendicular to the floor?   ○
8. Hands flat on the floor, fingers pointed forward?   ○
9. Head forward, cervical vertebrae in forward flexion with the chin tucked?   ○
10. Is the trainee breathing throughout?   ○
11. Does the trainee hold the final position for five full breath cycles?   ○

Cow

This is a simple hands-and-knees posture that uses upper, middle, and lower back muscle contraction to drive a stretch along the anterior shoulder and the lumbar and thoracic vertebrae. The cow reference comes from the sway back and head-up posture of cattle in the field.

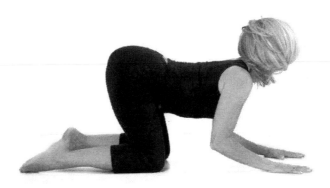

How to do it

1. Start in a kneeling position with the knees directly under the shoulders. The hips should be fully extended. The shins, tops of the feet, and toes should be in contact with the floor and point directly back (parallel to each other and perpendicular to the line of the shoulders).
2. Bend forward at the hips (flexion) and place the hands flat on the floor, fingers pointed directly forward. Slide the hands forward until both the arms and thighs are perpendicular to the floor.
3. In this intermediary "tabletop" position, the complete vertebral column should be in normal extension.

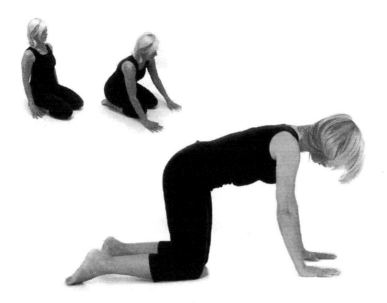

4. Execute a slow, powerful inhalation and contract the erector spinae muscles. Try to point the ischial tuberosities up. Pull the top of the pelvis up and the scapulae down and back as to meet. Squeeze the upper back musculature towards midline and lift the chest forward. Lift the head and look up towards the ceiling. This will combine to cause a dip in the center of the back (like a cow has). Bend (flex) the elbows, keeping them tucked in close to the body, and lower the torso halfway to the floor.
5. Return to the tabletop position by reacquiring normal extension of the vertebral column.
6. Repeat the sequence for five cycles.

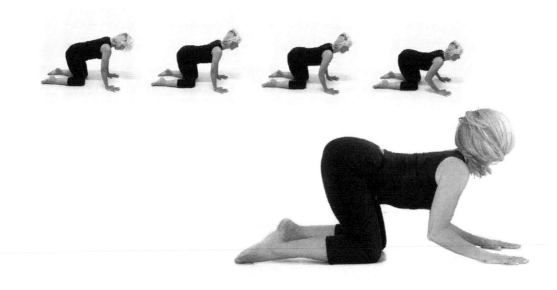

NOTE: After initial learning of the posture, this posture is a direct follow from the Cat posture. The positions directly alternate through the Tabletop posture without hesitation and without returning to the kneeling position.

What are the benefits?

1. A primary benefit is development of vertebral (lumbar and thoracic) range of motion through stretching of the anterior flexors (rectus abdominis, obliquus internus, obliquus externus).
2. Another primary benefit is development of shoulder range of motion through stretching of the anterior shoulder and thoracic musculature (pectoralis major, pectoralis minor, serratus anterior, intercostalis, subclavius).
3. In beginners, strength will be developed in the contracting posterior musculature.
4. When included as a part of a training sequence, this posture aids in the reduction of anxiety, depression, and perceived stress.
5. Develops local muscular endurance in all muscles actively contracting in the posture.

Contraindications

This is an extremely low risk posture. Individuals with diagnosed vertebral problems may want to avoid the posture or modify the degree of vertebral extension.

Learning and Teaching Checklist

1. Has the table top starting position been assumed correctly? ◯
2. Are the knees at approximately shoulder width? ◯
3. Are the knees, shins, ankles, tops of feet, and toes on the floor? ◯
4. Is the knee angle approximately 90°? ◯
5. Lumbar and thoracic back arched (in significant posterior extension)? ◯
6. Are the shoulders pulled back (scapulae retracted)? ◯
7. Are the arms perpendicular to the floor? ◯
8. Are the elbows bent and close to the torso? ◯
9. Are the hands flat on the floor, fingers pointed forward? ◯
10. Is the head facing up towards the ceiling? ◯
11. Is the trainee breathing throughout? ◯
12. Does the trainee hold the final position for five full breath cycles? ◯

Thread the Needle

~ Sucirandhrasana ~

This is a kneeling posture that develops range of motion at the shoulders. It also enhances rotational mobility of the vertebral column.

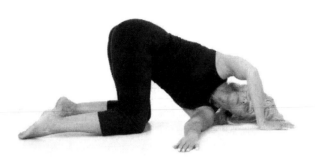

How to do it

1. Start in a kneeling position with the knees directly under the shoulders. The hips should be fully extended. The shins, tops of the feet, and toes should be in contact with the floor and point directly to the posterior (parallel to each other and perpendicular to the line of the shoulders).
2. Bend forward at the hips (flexion) and place the hands flat on the floor, fingers pointed directly forward. Slide the hands forward until both the arms and thighs are perpendicular to the floor.
3. In this intermediary "tabletop" position the complete vertebral column should be in normal extension.

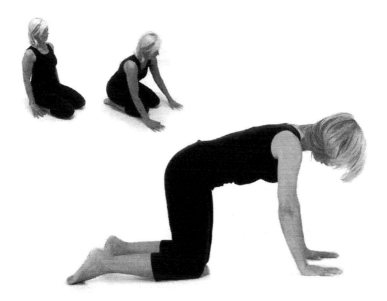

4. Slide one arm (now the lead) across the body, under and behind the other arm (now the trailing). In these illustrations, the lead side is the left side. Keep it straight and lower the lead shoulder to the floor as the arm crosses the body. The trailing elbow will bend (flex) to lower the torso.

5. Turn the head and torso to face as far to the trailing side as possible. Push on the trailing hand to keep the upper body position stable and to provide a gentle force to aid gravity in applying the stretch.

6. Rest the upper body's weight along the whole of the lead arm. Keep the lead palm up (supinate).

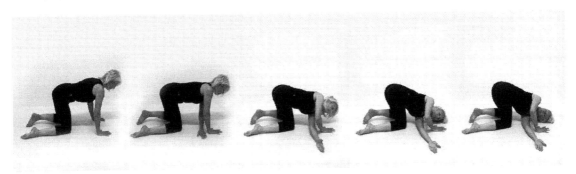

7. Extend the trailing leg and lift the knee. Stay on the trailing-foot toes and engage the abdominal musculature (navel to spine) for stability.
8. Now pronate the lead arm's hand so the palm is on the floor (for stability).

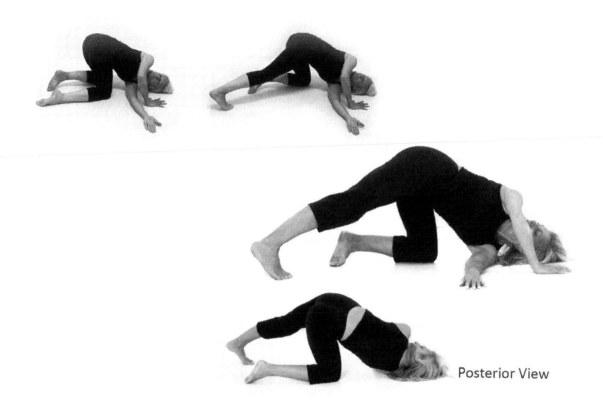

Posterior View

9. Hold for five breath cycles.
10. To exit, drop the knee and roll off the side of the forehead, pushing on the trailing palm to return to the table top position.

What are the benefits?

1. Provides a robust range of motion stimulus on the shoulder and back by stretching the posterior musculature (trapezius, latissimus dorsi, rhomboideus, serratus posterior, posterior deltoideus, quadratus lumborum).

2. Provides a controlled range of motion stimulus on the neck by providing a rotational stretch of the musculature (splenius capitus, levator scapulae, sternocleidomastoid, scalenus).
3. When included as a part of a training sequence, this posture aids in the reduction of anxiety, depression, and perceived stress.
4. Develops local muscular endurance in all muscles actively contracting in the posture.

Contraindications

Individuals with diagnosed cervical, vertebral, or shoulder problems may wish to avoid participation or employ a modification of the posture.

Learning and Teaching Checklist

1. Has the table top starting position been assumed correctly? ○
2. Knees initially approximately shoulder width apart? ○
3. Knees bent at approximately 90°? ○
4. Knees, shins, ankles, tops of feet, and toes on floor? ○
5. Shoulder on the floor, arm crossing under the body, behind the opposing arm, palm up? ○
6. Supporting arm bent and assisting the head and shoulders rotation to the end of their range of motion? ○
7. Is the trainee breathing throughout? ○
8. Does the trainee hold the final position for five full breath cycles? ○

"I've always found that anything worth achieving will always have obstacles in the way and you've got to have that drive and determination to overcome those obstacles on route to whatever it is that you want to accomplish."

Chuck Norris

Triplet 10

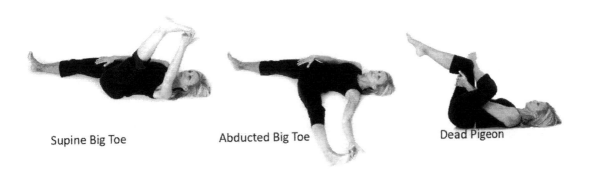

Supine Big Toe   Abducted Big Toe   Dead Pigeon

Supine Big Toe

~ Supta Padangusthasana ~

The Supine Big Toe posture is an effective developer of range of motion around the hip. This posture is frequently presented as part of a pair that includes the Abducted Big Toe posture.

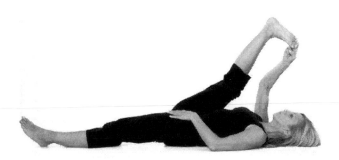

How to do it

1. Begin supine on the floor. The hands should be placed with the elbows touching the floor, palms directed upwards.

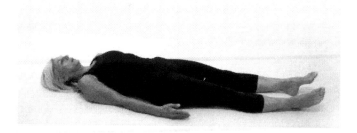

2. Bend one knee (the left in these illustrations) and bring the tigh to your chest. Hold it in place with the lead hand (same side) and pull gently to the chest.
3. Keep the hips level on the floor and the opposite leg (trailing leg) extended along the floor. Dorsiflex the toes (point towards the ceiling).

4. Place the trailing hand on the trailing leg, gently engaging the quadriceps to extend the trailing knee.
5. Hold behind the lead knee. Extend the knee. Point the toes toward your face (dorsiflex).
6. Wrap the first two fingers of the lead hand around the lead big toe. Beginners and those with poor flexibility will need to use a strap to create a connection between the foot and hand. Loop the strap just behind the ball of the foot. Alternatively, leave the hand behind the knee and work on extending the knee through quadriceps contraction and hamstrings relaxation.

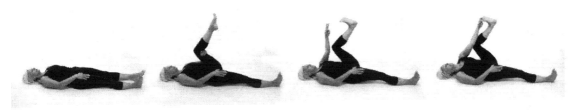

7. Extend the knee to full range of motion or to the limit of tolerance.

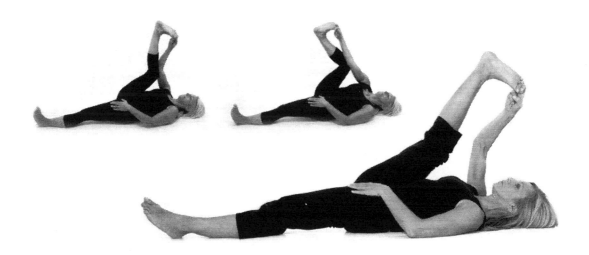

8. Hold for five breath cycles.
9. Release by bending the lead knee and then releasing the hand hold on the foot.
10. Lower the leg back to the original supine position.
11. Repeat the above process with the opposite leg.

NOTE: The next description in this triplet presents Supine Big Toe articulated in sequence with Abducted Big Toe. While Supine Big Toe can be done individually, one must assume the Supine Big Toe posture before entering into the Abducted Big to position.

What are the benefits?

1. Improves mobility (degree of flexion) around the hip.
2. It is composed of a gluteal & hamstring (semitendinosus, semimembranosus, and biceps femoris) stretch and a groin (adductor brevis, adductor longus, adductor magnus, pectineus, and gracilis) stretch. Beginners will also perceive a substantial calf (gastrocnemius, soleus, plantaris) stretch.
3. Reduces instances of low back pain.
4. When included as a part of a training sequence, this posture aids in the reduction of anxiety, depression, and perceived stress.
5. Develops local muscular endurance in all muscles actively contracting in the posture.

Contraindications

This is a very low risk posture. Although the risk is low, individuals with hypertension should be cautious if the immediately preceding posture was a standing posture; movement to a supine posture may aggravate orthostatic intolerance. Individuals with injuries, either acute or chronic, to the hamstrings should not participate in this posture.

Learning and Teaching Checklist

1. Is the toe grip correct?   ◯
2. Grip of toe precedes knee extension?   ◯
3. Are both hips in contact with the floor?   ◯
4. Is the trailing leg fully extended and in contact with the floor and one hand on top of the thigh?   ◯

5. Are the shoulders (not just the scapulae) and head in contact with the floor in full posture? ○
6. Is the lead leg's knee extended as dictated by ability and range of motion? ○
7. Is the trainee breathing throughout? ○
8. Does the trainee hold the final position for five full breath cycles? ○

Abducted Big Toe   ~ Continuation of Supta Padangusthasana ~

The Abducted Big Toe posture is a supine posture that develops range of motion around the hip. If this posture is included, it must follow the Supine Big Toe posture.

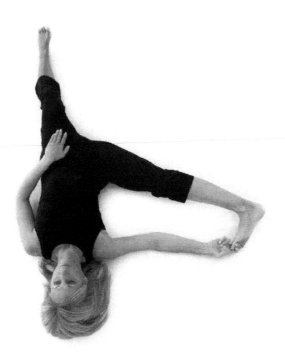

How to do it

1. Achieve the final position of the Supine Big Toe posture. Refer to the Supine Big Toe (above) for instructions on this initial step.

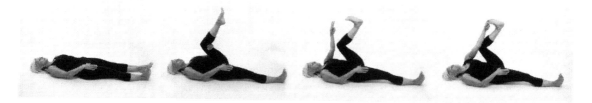

2. Extend the knee to full range of motion or the limit of tolerance and hold.

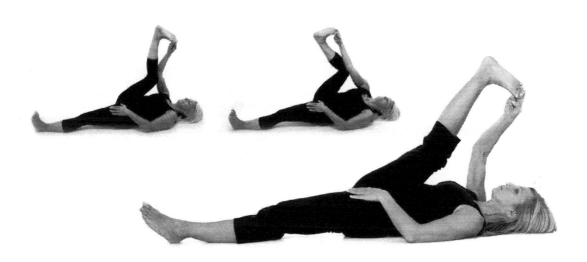

3. Abduct (lower) the leg laterally (outward to the side) to the floor or to the limit of movement.
4. Keep **both** hips on the floor (push down with the trailing hand to help cue this). Keep the knee on the floor in extension, and the toe pointed at the ceiling. These two points are imperative as they comprise the foundation of support and movement in this posture.
5. Keep pushing the lead heel out and away from the body.
6. Hold for five breath cycles.

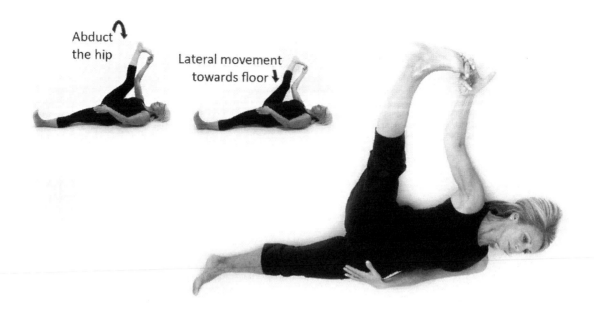

Abduct the hip

Lateral movement towards floor

7. Exit the posture by lifting the leg medially (inward to the middle) then bending the knee and releasing the hand hold on the foot.
8. Lower the leg back to the original supine position.
9. Repeat the above process for the opposite leg.

NOTE: When including this posture, it must follow the Supine Big Toe posture. It is not used as a stand-alone posture.

What are the benefits?

1. Improves mobility (degree of flexion and adduction) around the hip.
2. It is composed of a gluteal & hamstring (semitendinosus, semimembranosus, and biceps femoris) stretch during the assumption of the posture and a groin (adductor brevis, adductor longus, adductor magnus, pectineus, and gracilis) stretch during the posture. Beginners will also perceive a substantial calf (gastrocnemius, soleus, plantaris) stretch.
3. Reduces instances of low back pain.

4. When included as a part of a training sequence, this posture aids in the reduction of anxiety, depression, and perceived stress.
5. Develops local muscular endurance in all muscles actively contracting in the posture.

Contraindications

This is a low risk posture. Although the risk is low, individuals with hypertension should be cautious if the immediately preceding posture was a standing posture; movement to a supine posture may aggravate orthostatic intolerance. Individuals with injuries, either acute or chronic, to the hamstrings or adductors should not participate in this posture.

Learning and Teaching Checklist

1. Is the toe grip correct? ○
2. Grip of toe precedes knee extension? ○
3. Are both hips in contact with the floor throughout? ○
4. Trailing leg fully extended and in contact with the floor and one hand on top of the thigh? ○
5. Are the shoulders (not just the scapulae) and head in contact with the floor in full posture? ○
6. Is the lead leg's knee extended as dictated by ability and range of motion? ○
7. Lead leg abducted slowly away from midline with knee position and grip maintained? ○
8. Is the trainee breathing throughout? ○
9. Does the trainee hold the final position for five full breath cycles? ○

Dead Pigeon   ~ Supta Kapotasana ~

A stereotype commonly associated with yoga is the image of a hapless waif helplessly twisting themselves into a pretzel. This posture is the closest this book comes to that. The Dead Pigeon is a supine posture that primarily develops rotational range of motion at the hip. It also aids in developing abdominal muscle control. This position, unlike the stereotype, is easily achieved.

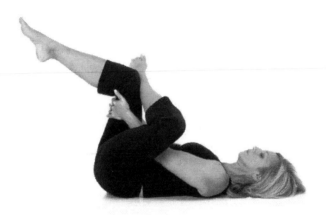

How to do it

1. Start in a lying position (Corpse) then bend your knees and draw your feet up towards the buttocks. The heels should be about one foot down from the ischial tuberosities.

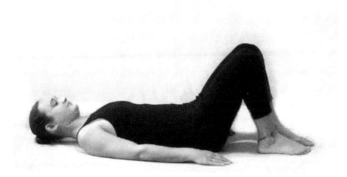

2. Flex the hip of the lead leg (right) so that the thigh approaches the chest.
3. Laterally rotate the femur so the shin of the lead leg crosses the body.
4. Place the ankle of the lead leg onto the thigh of the trailing leg about 4-6 inches above the knee. This may be an adequate end point for inducing a stretch in beginners. The shin of the lead leg should be approximately parallel to the floor.

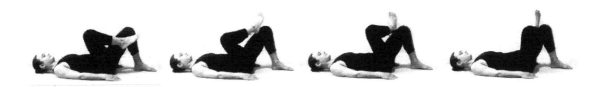

5. With the lead arm, reach through the space formed by the crossed legs. With the trailing arm, reach along the outside of the trailing leg (leg with foot flat on floor).
6. Lift the trailing leg off the floor by flexing at the hip until you can wrap both hands around the back of the trailing knee.
7. Pull gently and equally with the arms to bring the legs closer to the chest and to the end of the range of motion.
8. Keep the complete vertebral column in normal extension throughout the posture.

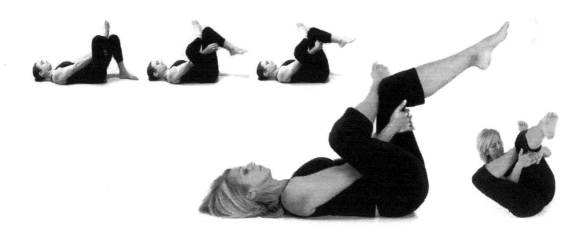

9. Hold for five breath cycles.
10. Reverse the process to exit and then repeat on the opposite side.

What are the benefits?

1. Improves mobility (degree of flexion and rotation) around the hip.
2. Acts as a stretch of the posterior hip musculature (semitendinosus, semimembranosus, and biceps femoris, gluteus maximus) and hip rotator muscles (piriformis, gemellus superior, gemellus inferior, obturator internus, obturator externus, and quadratus femoris).
3. Aids in developing abdominal musculature control.
4. Reduces instances of low back pain.
5. When included as a part of a training sequence, this posture aids in the reduction of anxiety, depression, and perceived stress.
6. Develops local muscular endurance in all muscles actively contracting in the posture.

Contraindications

This is a low risk posture. Although the risk is low, individuals with hypertension should be cautious if the immediately preceding posture was a standing posture; movement to a supine posture may aggravate orthostatic intolerance. Individuals with injuries, either acute or chronic, to the hips or knees should consider participation in this posture carefully.

Learning and Teaching Checklist

1. Both knees bent and then leading leg brought across? ○
2. Both hands grip around the back of the trailing knee? ○
3. Are both hips in contact with the floor throughout? ○
4. Is the leading leg's shin roughly parallel to floor? ○
5. Are the shoulders (not just the scapulae) and head in contact with the floor in full posture? ○
6. Are the legs pulled toward the chest as dictated by ability and range of motion? ○
7. Is the trainee breathing throughout? ○
8. Does the trainee hold the final position for five full breath cycles? ○

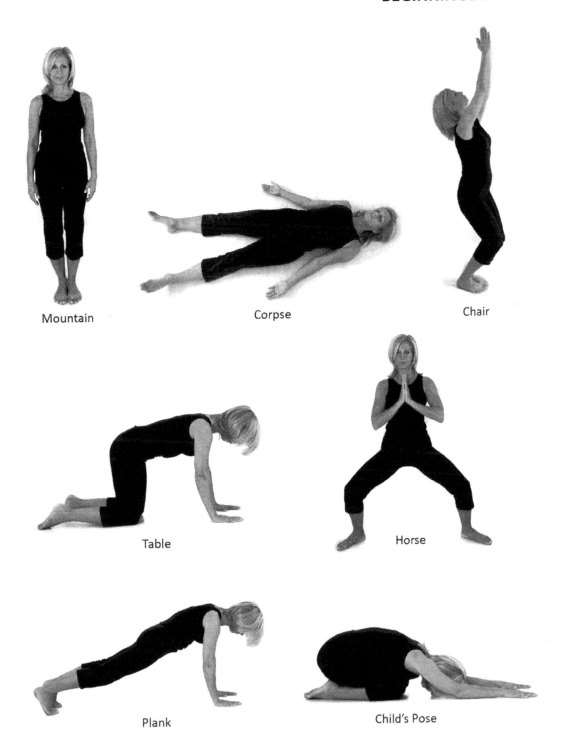

Mountain

Corpse

Chair

Table

Horse

Plank

Child's Pose

Mountain   ~ Tadasana ~

The Mountain Posture is a simple posture consisting of motionless standing. Correct standing posture is a basic health skill and in the context of yoga training it serves as an essential starting point for many individual yoga postures and as an intervening marker within a sequence of postures.

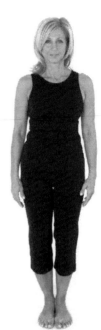

By starting in this position and returning to it after each standing posture, correct movement patterns can be developed. Isolating each subsequent standing posture by returning to the Mountain posture ensures that the correct motor patterns and sensations of balance are not affected by the preceding posture. By interjecting the Mountain posture between different postures, we are minimizing the effect of competing motor pathways and facilitating motor learning.

Although this is a low stress and non-taxing posture, it is important to adopt a fully upright anatomical position. This is a place where we can work on combatting the effects of days of hunching over a desk or PC or any other condition that leads to poor vertebral extension and carriage.

It is also important to "feel" ones balance in this posture and try to ensure that the center of pressure or balance is sensed at approximately mid-foot. Part of yoga is the development of balance and stability. Because we spend so much of our lives standing, it makes sense to ensure we are doing so in a mechanically correct manner.

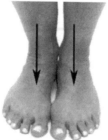

Equal pressure
on both feet

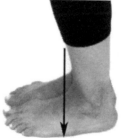

Center of Pressure
located at approximately
mid-foot

How to do it

1. Stand on the mat and assume a stance where the feet, ankles, and knees are together. For some individuals this may not be possible. In such cases, stand in as narrow a stance as possible. This narrow base of support helps develop balance and stability.

2. Stand fully erect and create an equivalent foundation where the center of balance or pressure is in the middle of each foot. You may want to gently rock forward onto the toes, backward onto the heels, and then gently forward again to find the desired point in the middle of the foot where you feel most balanced and stable.

3. The knees should be extended but not locked out agressively. They should also not be bent.

4. To control knee extension, gently engage the quadriceps (vastus medialis, vastus lateralis, vastus intermedus, and rectus femoris muscles above the knee) for stability.

5. Assume anatomically normal pelvic tilt. For many people the cue "tuck your tail bone under" or "lift your chest" will assist in this. At the same time, abdominal volume should be reduced through tensing the musculature. This is cued by saying "pull the navel back towards the vertebrae".

6. Raise the chest by vertebral extension in both the thoracic and lumbar vertebrae; "lengthen" your torso. This will feel like the distance between the lower ribs (costals) and hip bones (anterior iliac crest) has increased. If dealing with someone with poor posture or a weight problem, this simple postural change alone will make a small but visually noticeable change in appearance.

7. Ensure the cervical vertebrae (neck) are extended and the head is in a neutral position. It is useful to choose a landmark on the wall in front of the trainee at eye level as a focus spot. This will be helpful in maintaining correct head position. When done correctly the trainee will have a perception that the cervical spine has lengthened. You can use

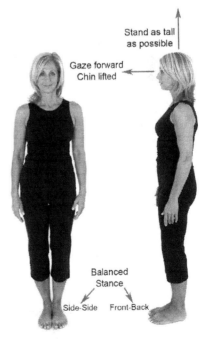

Stand as tall as possible

Gaze forward
Chin lifted

Balanced
Stance

Side-Side   Front-Back

this perception as a cue.

8. Once the body is aligned into the posture, it is often helpful to imagine a string pulling from the crown of the head upward to the ceiling.

9. During the time of the posture hold, attention should be on the body. We are attempting to exclude external stimulation and include only internal kinesthetic cues.

10. Maintenance of balance and stability is important here. Rescan the whole body frequently to ensure you have not rocked back onto the heels or toes. If you have, go back and use the process described in step one to find the center of the foot again. Some people will do this intuitively but others will require periodic reminders.

11. Hold for five breath cycles.

What are the benefits?

1. Development or reinforcement of anatomically correct posture.
2. Establishment of a root posture that aids in the transitions between different standing postures included in a yoga session.
3. Development or reinforcement of standing balance.
4. Improved motor control of postural musculature.
5. Improved attention and enhanced internal focus.
6. When included as a part of a training sequence, this posture aids in the reduction of anxiety, depression, and perceived stress.

Contraindications

For this position, there are no contraindications unless a pre-existing medical condition prevents standing. If an individual is not tolerant of orthostatic challenge (dizziness or loss of consciousness when moving from sit to stand or lying to stand) caution must be observed when returning from a posture to Mountain posture. In both of these latter instances a physician's clearance must be obtained prior to performing exercise.

Learning and Teaching Checklist

1. Is the body weight evenly distributed through both feet? ◯
2. Are knees extended but un-locked? ◯
3. Are the lordotic and kyphotic arches of the back held in normal extension

    (no excessive arching or rounding)? ⭕

4. Is the head held erect or is the chin tucked in? ⭕

5. Are the shoulders hunched forward or relaxed and back? ⭕

6. Are the arms hanging relaxed by the sides? ⭕

7. Is the trainee breathing throughout? ⭕

Chair

~ Utkatasana ~

This is a partial squat posture that develops the hip and knee musculature and can improve range of motion around the ankle. It also serves as a transition position for some postures.

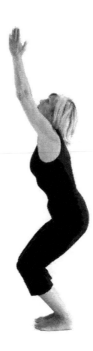

How to do it

1. Begin in Mountain posture and place the hands on the hips.
2. Press the ankles, calves, and knees together to establish a stable position.
3. Slowly flex (bend) the hips and knees. The hips should move back slightly and the knees should move forward in front of the toes. The body weight should be spread evenly across the feet. There should be a sense of muscular tension in the lower extremities.
4. Engage the abdominal musculature. You should feel like you are attempting to pull your navel back towards the vertebral column.
5. The cervical spine should be in normal extension with head and eyes facing directly to the front.

6. Raise the hands above the head, elbows extended as much as possible, biceps facing the ears, and palms together if possible.

7. Squeeze the shoulder blades together (retract the scapulae towards midline). Slightly bend (unlock) the elbows to allow the shoulders to relax down and back (this is driven by gravity not contraction). Gently roll the head back into cervical extension and look at the thumbs.

8. In the final position, the torso should be relatively upright and the angle between the femur (thigh) and tibia (shin) should be approximately 100° to 120°.

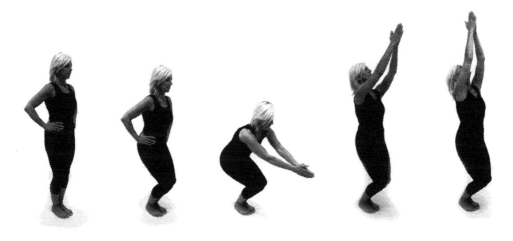

9. Hold for five breath cycles.

What are the benefits?

1. Develops local muscular endurance in the gluteals, quadriceps (rectus femoris, vastus medialis, vastus lateralis, vastus internus), and the posterior calf muscles (gastrocnemius, soleus, plantaris).

2. In beginners, develops strength in the gluteals, quadriceps (rectus femoris, vastus medialis, vastus lateralis, vastus internus), and the posterior calf muscles (gastrocnemius, soleus, plantaris).

3. Improves standing posture.

4. When included as a part of a training sequence, this posture aids in the reduction of anxiety, depression, and perceived stress.

5. Develops local muscular endurance in all muscles actively contracting in the posture.

Contraindications

This is a low risk posture as it presents no orthostatic challenge. There is increased vascular resistance to blood flow via raised arms that might be of concern to someone with diagnosed heart disease. As there are no rotational and extremely limited shear stresses, this is a knee-safe posture.

Learning and Teaching Checklist

1. Is the bodyweight evenly spread across the feet (equal body mass in front and behind mid-foot)?
2. Are the knees forward?
3. Are the hips slightly back?
4. Is the torso mostly upright (no more than a small lean forward)?
5. Is the line of sight directed upward?
6. Are the arms extended overhead with palms facing together?
7. Is the trainee breathing throughout?
8. Does the trainee hold the final position for five full breath cycles?

Horse Stance   ~ No equivalent Sanskrit ~

This posture originated in the martial arts as a means to establish a base of stability when in combat on boats or other unstable surfaces. The Horse stance is a simple posture that develops range of motion laterally around the hips and loads the quadriceps and gluteals. It can serve as an excellent transition position, used instead of the Mountain posture for more advanced trainees who desire a more rigorous endurance training stimulus.

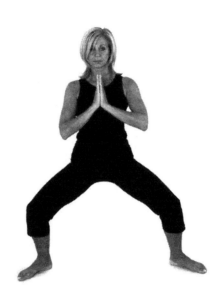

How to do it

1. Begin in Mountain posture.
2. Flex (bend) the elbows to 45- 90°, extend the hands backwards at the wrist, place the palms together in front of the body, and raise both arms up until the thumbs are resting on the sternum.
3. Step with the right foot laterally. This should be a wide step, approximately three to four feet depending on leg length.

4. Point the toes out (rotate the whole leg so the knees and toes are pointing the same direction) to about 45°. As ability increases over time, so should foot width, in order to continue providing a stretching stimulus.

5. Squat down to a point where the top of the thighs are just above parallel to the floor and keep the torso as close to vertical as possible (chest up). The knees should be pushed out so the femurs are along the same 45° angle as the feet.

6. Keep the lumbar, thoracic, and cervical vertebrae in normal extension with the head held neutral and eyes forward.

7. It is important to push the pelvis forward in order to produce the desired inner thigh stretch and knee dominant musculature loading. If the hips are allowed to push back, inner thigh tension is lost and the loading shifts to hip dominance. Note that when the hips move forward, the knees will too. This is fine.

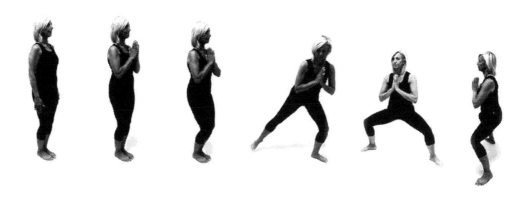

8. Hold for five breath cycles.

What are the benefits?

1. One of the primary benefits is improved balance control.

2. Improved lateral range of motion around the hips through stretching of the adductors (adductor brevis, adductor longus, adductor magnus, pectineus, and gracilis).

3. In beginners, improved strength in the quadriceps (rectus femoris, vastus lateralis, vastus medialis, vastus intermedus), abductors (sartorius, tensor fascia latae), and gluteals.

4. When included as a part of a training sequence, this posture aids in the reduction of anxiety, depression, and perceived stress.
5. Develops local muscular endurance in all muscles actively contracting in the posture.

Contraindications

This is a low risk posture. Those with diagnosed hip joint problems may wish to avoid participation or modify the posture.

Learning and Teaching Checklist

1. Is the bodyweight distributed evenly across soles of the feet?   ○
2. Are the legs holding a wide stance with foot angle of 45° or greater?   ○
3. Does the angle of the thighs match the angle of feet?   ○
4. Is the torso vertical with the chest lifted?   ○
5. Are the arms in front, palms together, fingertips at the level of the chin?   ○
6. Is the head facing directly forward?   ○
7. Is the trainee breathing throughout?   ○
8. Does the trainee hold the final position for five full breath cycles?   ○

Table Posture & Child's Pose   ~ No Sanskrit Equivalent & Balnasana ~

The Table Posture and Child's Pose are closely related kneeling postures that can be used as entry and exit postures or as intermediary positions linking postures where the body is supported on the hands and feet. They can also be used as rest or recovery positions for beginning individuals who cannot stay in postures like Up Dog, Down Dog, or Plank for the recommended duration.

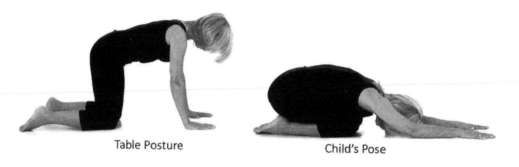

Table Posture   Child's Pose

How to do it

1. Begin in a hands and knees position on the floor.
2. The hands should be directly under the shoulders and the hips directly over the knees. The toes should be pointed directly backwards with the tops of the feet and shins on the floor).
3. The head should be facing the floor. The neck should be in normal extension.
4. This position is called the Table Posture.
5. Flex at the knees and move the ischial tuberosities (butt bones) back until they are resting on the heels (calcaneous bones of both feet). This will place your feet at roughly hip width.

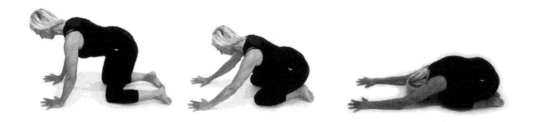

6. Stretch the arms straight forward on the ground, palms down, as far as you can reach. The hands should be directly in front of the shoulder joints (not too narrow or too wide). Spread the fingers; this improves area of floor contact and helps ensure stability.
7. Arch the lower back (keep it as straight as possible).
8. The forehead should be facing the floor or resting on the floor.

What are the benefits?

1. The Child's Pose develops range of motion around the hip by stretching the hamstrings and range of motion around the shoulder joint.
2. Combined, the postures aid in developing kinaesthetic awareness and lumbar back control.
3. The Child's Pose can promote a sensation of relaxation.
4. When included as a part of a training sequence, these postures aid in the reduction of anxiety, depression, and perceived stress.

Contraindications

These are low risk postures. Those with diagnosed hip and knee joint problems may wish to avoid participation. Individuals with shoulder extension problems may wish to refrain from or modify the Child's Pose.

Learning and Teaching Checklist

1. Initially, when in Table posture, is a hands-and-knees posture assumed?　　○
2. Are the hands directly under the shoulders and the knees directly under the hips?　　○
3. Are the Fingers pointed forward and are the toes pointed to the rear?　　○
4. Are the knees bent at approximately 90°?　　○
5. Is the neck in normal extension and the head not looking up or down excessively?　　○
6. In the transition to the Child's Pose, do the hips sink back toward the heels as far as possible?　　○
7. Are the shoulders in full extension with the lower back arched, elbows fully extended, and fingers spread wide?　　○

8. Is the trainee breathing throughout? ◯
9. Does the trainee hold the final position for five full breath cycles? ◯

Plank   ~ Kumbhakasana ~

The plank is a suspended posture that strongly develops midline stability throughout the entire long axis of the body. It can be used as both a primary posture and a transitional posture.

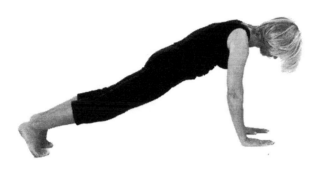

How to do it

1. Starting in the Standing Forward Fold posture, step back approximately 2.5 – 3 feet (depending on leg length) with one foot. This foot is now the trailing foot. Bend the opposite (now the lead) leg to make this transition. Follow on by moving the lead foot beside the trailing foot. Keep the heels up off the floor.
2. The arms and hands should be directly under the shoulders and the scapulae should be retracted and depressed (pulled together and down towards the hips).
3. Externally rotate the arms. This will point the elbows out and back and will require the scapulae to be rotated medially and squeezed towards midline.

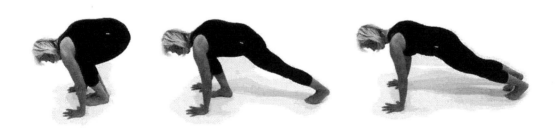

4. Lift the chest to ensure that the thoracic and lumbar curves are held in normal extension.
5. The abdominal musculature (rectus abdominis, external obliques, transversus abdominis) should be tensed to add rigidity from the shoulders down to the hips.
6. Engage the quadriceps and extend the knees in order to achieve a straight line from the shoulder joint down to the ankles.
7. The neck (cervical vertebrae) should be in normal extension keeping the head and eyes facing the floor about a foot in front of the hands.

What are the benefits?

1. The primary outcome of practicing the Plank is a substantial improvement in midline stability.
2. The isometric contraction of such a large mass of muscle also creates a metabolic training effect that contributes to local muscular endurance development.
3. In beginning trainees, strengthens the muscles supporting the arches of the feet, the knees, hips, vertebrae, shoulders, elbows, wrist, and hands.
4. Improves standing posture.
5. When included as a part of a training sequence, this posture aids in the reduction of anxiety, depression, and perceived stress.
6. Develops local muscular endurance in all muscles actively contracting in the posture.

Contraindications

The primary issue preventing participation in this posture is any wrist or hand pathology such as carpal tunnel syndrome or advanced arthritis.

Learning and Teaching Checklist

1. Are the arms and hands directly under the shoulders? ◯
2. Is the bodyweight supported on the palms of the hands and the balls of the feet? ◯
3. Is the body straight along its long axis (ankles, knees, hips, shoulders in line)? ◯
4. Is the upper back not rounded? ◯
5. Is the head not drooping? ◯

6. Is the trainee breathing throughout? ○

7. Does the trainee hold the final position for five full breath cycles? ○

Corpse

~ Shavasana ~

Simply lying down reduces the vertical distance the heart has to pump blood and the work it has to do. Lying down also supports all parts of the body and removes postural muscular effort. This supine posture, deriving its name from the position of a cadaver on a coroner's table, traditionally concludes every yoga session. The intent is to provide an effortless position that facilitates recovery, relaxation, and reflection. It is often accompanied by sensory and environmental aids to relaxation.

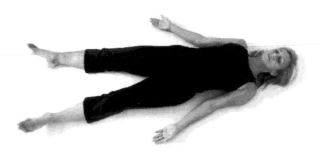

How to do it

1. The trainee will just have transitioned from a close-to-the-floor posture and will assume a supine position (lying on their back) on the mat.
2. Close your eyes.
3. The feet should be spread apart to where they are about hip width, the toes pointing slightly to the outside (laterally).
4. The knees and hips should be in normal extension.
5. The lumbar region should be relaxed and in normal extension.
6. The bodyweight of the torso should be spread across the thoracic region.
7. The scapulae (shoulder blades) should be gently retracted (squeezed slightly together) so they rest flat on the mat. Gently lift one shoulder blade off the mat, rotate the shoulder around, back and down. Now do the other.
8. The neck should be in normal extension, with the chin tucked, head facing directly at the ceiling and resting on the occipital bone.
9. The arms should have the elbows fully but softly extended, the palms face up. Angle the arms slightly away from the body (somewhere between 15° and 45°) from the

long axis of the body. Legs and arms too close to the midline of the body slow body cooling, too far away cause bending and compression of blood vessels and increase resistance to blood flow.

10. All muscles and joints should be released of any tension. If the instructor's purpose of this section is to create relaxation and contemplation then use of a light cover, blanket, or towel would be appropriate to make the posture comfortable for a longer period.

What are the benefits?

1. Provides post-session recovery via a decreased heart rate and respiratory rate.
2. Creates a sensation of deep relaxation.
3. When included as a part of a training sequence, this posture aids in the reduction of anxiety, depression, and perceived stress.

Contraindications

There are no contraindications to this posture as it is non-exertional.

Learning and Teaching Checklist

1. Is the trainee lying down? ○
2. Are the feet approximately hip width? ○
3. Are all the elements of the axial skeleton held in normal (neutral) extension? ○
4. Are the arms slightly away from the body with elbows extended and palms up? ○
5. Are the eyes closed? ○
6. Does the trainee feel relaxed? ○
7. Is the trainee breathing throughout? ○

"A little nonsense, now and then, is relished by the wisest men."

Willy Wonka

YOGA RESOURCES

Further Instruction

Comprehensive Yoga Teacher Training – seasonalyoga.co.uk
Practicing Teacher Support – seasonalyogaonline.com
Specialized Anatomy Workshops for Teachers – yoganatomy.com
Yoga Practice Workshops and Apps – johnscottyoga.com
Online Introduction to Yoga Instruction – yogawod.org
Online Course in Physiology for Fitness Professionals – physiologywod.org
Online Courses in Anatomy for Fitness Professionals – anatomywod.org

Personal Equipment

Yoga Mats, Towels, and Blocks – gaiam.com
Yoga Mats, Towels, and Blocks – manduka.com
Yoga Mats, Towels, and Blocks – lululemon.com
Yoga Mats, Towels, and Blocks – amazon.com
Yoga Mats, Towels – walmart.com
Yoga Mats, Towels – asda.com

Clothing

Women's Yoga Fashion – lululemon.com
Women's Yoga Fashion – sweatybetty.com
Men's Yoga Fashion – prana.com
Men's and Women's Yoga Appropriate Clothing – amazon.com
Men's and Women's Yoga Appropriate Clothing – walmart.com
Men's and Women's Yoga Appropriate Clothing – asda.com

The Authors

Julie Hanson – juliehanson.com
Lon Kilgore – lonkilgore.com

"It matters little how much equipment we use;
it matters much that we be masters of all we do use."

Sam Abell

ANATOMICAL GLOSSARY

Directions

Anterior – toward the front
Posterior – toward the back
Superior – toward the head
Inferior – toward the feet
Medial – toward the midline, in the middle
Lateral – away from the midline, to the side
Proximal – closer to midline
Distal – farther from midline

Body Regions

Cervical – refers to the neck, defined by the vertebrae above those attaching to the ribs and below the skull
Thoracic – a space or area of the trunk of the body above the diaphragm (at the base of the ribs) and also refers to the vertebrae attaching to the ribs.
Lumbar – refers to an area of the back defined by the vertebrae below the ribs and above the hips (pelvis)
Abdominal – a space or area of the trunk of the body below the diaphragm and ending at the top of the pelvic bones
Kyphosis – normal curve of the upper back, or the kyphotic curve
Lordosis – normal curve of the lower back, or lordotic curve

Movements

Flexion – bending of a joint to make its angle smaller (like closing a book)
Extension – bending of a joint to make its angle larger (like opening a book)
Rotation – revolving of a joint or body part around an axis (like a wheel on an axle)
Abduction – moving a body part away from the body (like opening a car door)
Adduction – moving a body part toward the body (like closing a car door)
Dorsiflexion – pointing the toes upward (lift the toes off the floor with heels down)
Plantarflexion – pointing the toes downward (lift the heels off the floor with toes down)

Bones

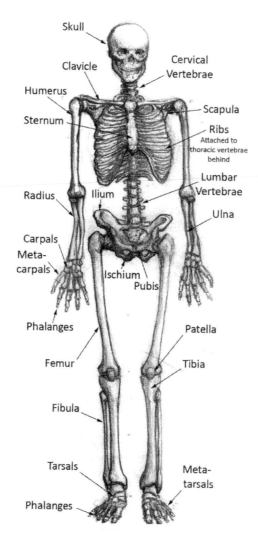

General reference for locations of bones

Basic Muscles

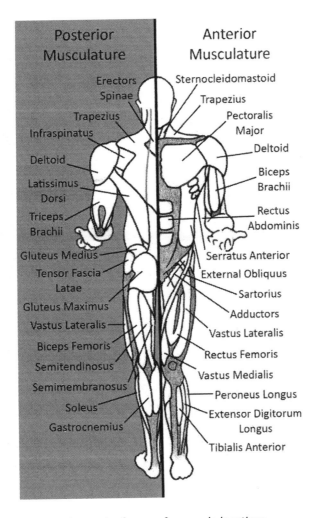

Posterior Musculature — Anterior Musculature

Erectors Spinae
Trapezius
Infraspinatus
Deltoid
Latissimus Dorsi
Triceps Brachii
Gluteus Medius
Tensor Fascia Latae
Gluteus Maximus
Vastus Lateralis
Biceps Femoris
Semitendinosus
Semimembranosus
Soleus
Gastrocnemius

Sternocleidomastoid
Trapezius
Pectoralis Major
Deltoid
Biceps Brachii
Rectus Abdominis
Serratus Anterior
External Obliquus
Sartorius
Adductors
Vastus Lateralis
Rectus Femoris
Vastus Medialis
Peroneus Longus
Extensor Digitorum Longus
Tibialis Anterior

General reference for muscle locations

Abdominals – Generic term for the Rectus Abdominis, External Obliques, and Internal Obliques muscles of the anterior and lateral abdomen

Adductors – Generic term for the Adductor Brevis, Adductor Longus, Adductor Magnus, and Adductor Minimus muscles of the medial hip

Calves – Generic term for the Gastrocnemius and Soleus muscles of the lower leg (also known as the Triceps Surae)

Hamstrings – Generic term for the Semitendinosus, Semimembranosus, and Biceps Femoris muscles of the posterior thigh

Quadriceps – Generic term for the Vastus Medialis, Vastus Intermedius, Vastus Lateralis, and Rectus Femoris of the anterior thigh

"People rarely succeed unless they have fun in what they are doing."

Dale Carnegie